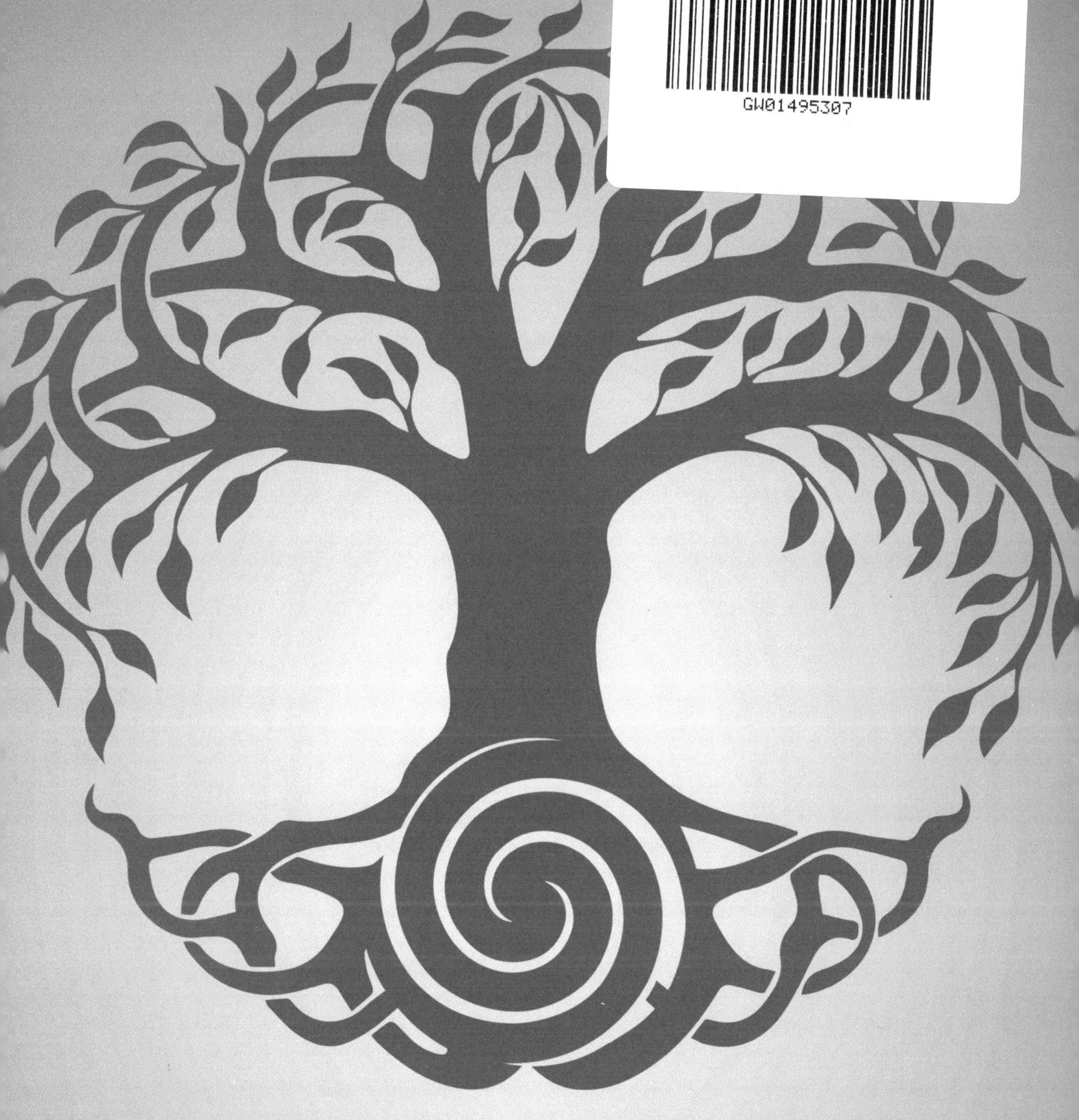

Holistic Cognitive Behaviour Therapy

A strengths-based approach integrating body, mind and spirit within the wider context

Dr Hilary Garraway

Pavilion

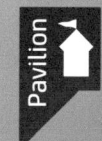

Holistic Cognitive Behaviour Therapy

A strengths-based approach integrating body, mind and spirit within the wider context

© Pavilion Publishing & Media

The author has asserted her rights in accordance with the Copyright, Designs and Patents Act (1988) to be identified as the author of this work.

Published by:
Pavilion Publishing and Media Ltd
Blue Sky Offices
25 Cecil Pashley Way
Shoreham by Sea
West Sussex
BN43 5FF

Tel: 01273 434 943
Email: info@pavpub.com
Web: www.pavpub.com

Published 2021
All rights reserved. No part of this publication may be reproduced, stored in a retrieval system, or transmitted in any form or by any means, electronic, mechanical, photocopying, recording or otherwise, without prior permission in writing of the publisher and the copyright owners.

A catalogue record for this book is available from the British Library.

ISBN: 978-1-914010-60-6

Pavilion Publishing and Media is a leading publisher of books, training materials and digital content in mental health, social care and allied fields. Pavilion and its imprints offer must-have knowledge and innovative learning solutions underpinned by sound research and professional values.

Authors: Dr Hilary Garraway
Production editor: Mike Benge, Pavilion Publishing and Media Ltd
Cover design: Emma Dawe, Pavilion Publishing and Media Ltd
Page layout and typesetting: Anthony Pitt, Pavilion Publishing and Media Ltd
Printing: Halstan & Co Ltd

Contents

About the author 1

Acknowledgments 2

Foreword 3

Introduction 7

Chapter 1: A Holistic approach to CBT 17

Chapter 2: The holistic CBT model 45

Chapter 3: Our human spirit 67

Chapter 4: The HCBT developmental model 93

Chapter 5: HCBT as an individual therapy 107

Chapter 6: The process of HCBT 117

Epilogue 145

References 150

Other titles from Pavilion Publishing 157

About the author

Dr Hilary Garraway BSc. MSc. DClinPsych CPsychol is a consultant clinical psychologist and BABCP-accredited CBT therapist, supervisor and trainer. She works full time as an adult psychology lead in Barnet, Enfield and Haringey Mental Health Trust, and before that she worked in Early Intervention in Psychosis teams. Hilary has been a therapist for over 30 years and has worked in the NHS for about 20 years, as well as a range of settings including residential child care, youth and community work and the voluntary sector. She has trained in person-centred art therapy, ecotherapy, spiritual direction and creative writing. Hilary also trained as an adult education teacher and is an honorary lecturer at University College London, University of Hertfordshire and King's College London. She has been a trustee for various charities and is currently a trustee for two charities that develop whole person health care, and is the former chair of the National Spirituality and Mental Health Forum and former British Psychological Society spirituality lead.

Hilary has a special interest in psychospiritual development and integrating spirituality into therapy and describes her spirituality as Celtic and contemplative within the Christian tradition. Together with her husband who is originally from Grenada, she has set up a charity there and they are in the process of establishing a therapeutic retreat house in Grenada. They have two adult children and a labradoodle dog.

Acknowledgments

In memory of Stuart Bowtell, whose terminal illness in the prime of his young life started me questioning and which led me to a deeper spiritual journey.

Also in memory of Dr Mike Sheldon, whose work and passion for whole person health care set the foundations for my journey towards Holistic CBT.

I wish to thank Bernard Cope for the drawings of the HCBT model and formulations, to Hayley Garraway for redrawing the tree for chapter 2, and to those who gave permission for their material to be used in the case examples provided.

Foreword

The Cognitive behavioural therapy (CBT) approach can be summarised as *'What we think affects how we feel and what we do'*. At times when people become distressed they tend to fall into repeating patterns of unhelpful thinking (with self-blame, negative views of themselves, their situation and the future), and unhelpful actions or behaviours (such as reduced activity, avoidance or unhelpful responses such as pushing others away, taking risks or drinking to excess). The classic CBT approach helps to understand the person here and now, using the problem-focused model.

CBT is evidence based and widely recommended. But it is not without criticism - often focused on three main issues:

i. That the way much CBT has been delivered can seem overly manualised and structured - overly emphasising the *structure* of therapy over the therapeutic *relationship*.

ii. It's focus on *here and now* current problems may overlook the importance of the past and personal/developmental history.

iii. It's focus is on the individual problems - ignores the wider social network and systemic factors in the person's life such as relationships, job loss, poverty and debt.

That is where Holistic cognitive behavioural therapy (HCBT) is so helpful. It focuses on the developing thinking of inclusivity and person-centred CBT to emphasise the importance of beliefs, personal meanings and relationships. It includes the importance individuals place on their own spiritual or personal faith traditions, or none, in addition to the everyday negative automatic thoughts and schemas that are the bread and butter of CBT. As such it brings a breath of fresh air to CBT working by giving permission for patients to discuss freely any aspects of their own life - including spiritual concerns or supports that can be often overlooked in a more traditional mental health formulation.

Professor Aaron Beck - one of the developers of the CBT approach claims that CBT can act as *The Integrative Therapy* and can incorporate other therapeutic approaches. This strong argument is perhaps made because the CBT model argues that when someone feels better it is because fundamental changes have occurred in their thoughts and behaviours. HCBT can be seen as a powerful resource to broaden self-understanding - and aid recovery. It does this by achieving that other key goal of CBT - to help people become their own therapist and thereby contribute to their own ongoing healing. The book cleverly draws on the range of so-called third wave CBT therapies that have developed over the last two decades. At the same time, it uses a non-judgemental language that frees the patient to express their own opinions, beliefs, hopes and fears and normalises these discussions for use within professional settings in the NHS, social care and beyond. It not only expands assessment by taking a flexible transtheoretical approach that looks beyond the individual, but also includes important concepts such as ecotherapy, ecology and climate change. Climate fear is increasingly an issue for younger and older people who value Green/ecological issues and see these as a central part of their self-identify. The current Climate Crisis can lead many to experience feelings of hopelessness and powerlessness in the face of forces that individuals alone feel they cannot address. Climate remains little mentioned or focused upon in traditional CBT assessment and training models and it is a welcome added focus to this book.

The course is written by a trained and accredited CBT practitioner and practicing Consultant Clinical Psychologist. It uses the widely applied and evidence-based CBT framework, but cleverly modified to emphasise meaning, acceptance, compassion and mindful elements and the use of concepts of spirit to provide a holistic view of self. These different elements remind practitioners that people's world views can be complicated, and that helping them make sense of why they feel as they do, and plan a way out of distress requires a personal narrative and formulation that makes sense to them and addresses the full range of concerns and priorities they see as important. To work in this way requires sensitive enquiry that is always focused on the beliefs of the patient rather than the assumptions and prior expectations of the therapist. A holistic approach provides a structure for trained CBT therapists to safely help people explore their beliefs and experiences in a holistic way, and to do this in an ethical and professional way. The linked training manual, *'Free to be Me'* is to be welcomed and encourages users of the book to familiarise themselves with the approach and teach others if they wish. It is at this point I would add a proviso. CBT - and Holistic CBT should be delivered and taught by practitioners who are already competent and trained in CBT. The book and resources are not suited for people without CBT experience. I would encourage anyone who is enthused to offer the course to seek CBT training and accreditation first, or to jointly deliver the course with someone who has these skills.

I hope readers find the concepts in the book raise interesting and challenging questions about their practise, inclusivity, use of accessible language and models of engagement. It will hopefully empower therapists to focus on a wider range of thoughts, fears and responses than have been conventionally asked. I encourage you to take the bits that broaden your work and thinking and try them out. Experiment and discover with your patients what they find helpful, then integrate that learning into your own practice. Use these broader concepts and integrate what you learn with your own personality and communication skills to develop your own Holistic CBT. It promises to be a fascinating journey.

Professor Chris Williams MBChB BSc MMedSc MD FRCPsych Hon Fellow BABCP

Emeritus Professor of Psychosocial Psychiatry, University of Glasgow, a Past - President of the British Association for Behavioural and Cognitive Psychotherapies (BABCP) and lead author of the widely used Living Life to the Full approach (www.llttf.com).

Introduction

This book is the culmination of my journey so far in developing Holistic CBT (Cognitive Behaviour Therapy). It draws on both my personal and professional journey of seeking to be more integrated and whole as a person, as well as on the experiences I have had helping others in their journeys with mental health and well-being. It does not set out to be an academic textbook though I will refer to some of the literature that has helped me and I will reference literature and research should you wish to dig deeper. These references can act as signposts to those readers who wish to explore the academic side more fully. This work has not grown out of academic research with carefully controlled trials but from the raw day-to-day clinical work of secondary adult mental health care. My focus has always been a pragmatic approach and my aim is to offer a tool that can be used in various settings with a range of people. So, my motivation is seeing what works in practice and this book is very much a practical book to help people use Holistic CBT (HCBT).

This book sets out the HCBT model so that, along with the *Free to Be Me* manual, it will enable others to use HCBT in their own work and in particular to run the 'Free to be Me' course, based on this HCBT model.

HCBT has grown out of my therapeutic work with the NHS and this book is written for health and social care professionals as well as staff in the voluntary sector, faith groups, community organisations and anyone who is working therapeutically with clients. Some of you may have life experience of mental health issues and some of you may have skills and training in areas such as counselling and group work. Whoever you are, thank you for reading this book and considering the possibility of using HCBT and running the Free to be Me course.

I have seen the benefits that the course has brought and so this book offers another tool you can use in your own work to improve the lives of others. I want this book to reach a wide audience and not just be for health care professionals, and for that reason I have sought to avoid psychological terminology or theoretical language where possible. However, a basic understanding of standard CBT would be very useful to have before reading this book, and particularly before running the Free to be Me course. I have therefore listed some recommended reading at the end of this chapter which will offer a good introduction to CBT.

The goal of HCBT is to develop the person rather than to solve a problem or simply reduce symptoms. By having this focus, it is not only for those who have diagnosed mental health symptoms but for anyone who wants to develop themselves as a person. In focusing on who a person is and exploring what is important to them, then symptoms can decrease or goals can be achieved despite their symptoms. Free to be Me is therefore as much a personal development course as it is a course to reduce mental health symptoms.

The course itself has been used by a wide range of people – from those who have been long-term clients of secondary mental health services including those who have had inpatient admissions, to those who are functioning well and have never needed mental health services. I have run it in NHS secondary care mental health settings as part of therapeutic care, as well as running it within a community setting as a personal development course. It has also been run online using a video conferencing tool, which opens up the possibility of running the course for a group of participants from a wide range of cultural backgrounds and geographic locations. It is hoped that it will be run in many more varied places over time. It has been particularly useful for those who want to learn more about themselves or those who feel they have little sense of self. The course can also be helpful for people who feel at a crossroads in life, unclear where they are heading and unsure of any sense of meaning and purpose in their life.

I have been hesitant to put pen to paper (or more accurately fingertip to keyboard) but, as a good friend said to me before I started writing this book, it is better to do something imperfectly than to do nothing perfectly. So this book outlines my thinking so far and highlights the different influences that have shaped that thinking. HCBT is a patchwork of different ideas and many you will recognise from different CBT practices, but hopefully there will be a few things that are new to you, too. I will try and give credit to ideas when I know the source but I am aware that a lot of things in this book are drawn from common CBT practices and from other therapies which won't be referenced, so I apologise in advance to those whose ideas I have used without referencing. CBT is like baking a cake: there are some standard ingredients which are necessary and then there are numerous variations of the basic CBT recipe. I hope that I'm offering something that is in some ways familiar but which also has a new twist to the recipe and a few extra ingredients to spice up the mix!

I am very aware that this is an ongoing journey of discovery and I am always reading more and learning from others. Each time I run the course there are changes I make. This book is not therefore a sign that I am totally satisfied with where I have got to, but is more a pause on my journey at a point where the changes are minimal enough to put it in print. But I also hope that in sharing it with you, I gain some feedback if you run the course or use the material in other ways. I'm interested to learn from others on similar journeys so I welcome any feedback or reflections that this book may prompt in you.

In developing a holistic model there is always more to add and different aspects of the model to develop, so by publishing this book I hope that HCBT will continue to grow and be shaped by those who use it.

Holisim

Let me start by explaining what I mean by 'holistic' because it can mean different things to different people. The term 'holism' was first used by the naturalist J.C. Smuts referring to 'the fundamental factor operative towards the creation of wholes in the universe' (Smuts, 1927).

Aristotle offered a useful definition of holism when he famously said that 'the sum is greater than its parts'. From the same era there is the following aspect of holism which is integral to the HCBT model, as quoted from Plato:

> 'As you ought not to attempt to cure the eyes without the head, or the head without the body, so neither ought you to attempt to cure the body without the soul . . . for the part can never be well unless the whole is well.' (Phaedrus, as quoted in Ross, 1997)

So when I refer to Holistic CBT I am talking about seeing the whole person in their whole context and seeking to work with all aspects of a person. I considered using the term 'whole person', and apart from the fact it doesn't roll off the tongue as easily as holistic, for me 'whole person' doesn't capture everything that needs to be included. 'Whole person' implies that the focus is all *within* the person, rather than including the wider context as well. As you will see, HCBT is as much about a person's context and the connectivity with this context as it is about the internal factors of the individual, hence my choice of the word 'holistic'.

Holism also encapsulates something about balance and holding opposites in tension. This for me brings to mind the concepts of ying and yang, of left and right hemispheres of the brain, of the physical and the spiritual, and about seeking wholeness by bringing different aspects into balance. Holism implies integration and balance between different aspects of ourselves. Dan Siegel, a clinical professor of psychiatry, described a river of integration flowing between one river bank which is chaos, and the other which is rigidity, saying:

> 'Integration enables us to be flexible and free; the lack of such connections promotes a life that is either rigid or chaotic, stuck and dull on the one hand or explosive and unpredictable on the other. With the connecting freedom of integration comes a sense of vitality and the ease of well-being. Without integration we can become imprisoned in behavioural ruts – anxiety and depression, greed, obsession, and addiction.' (Siegel, 2010)

The term holistic has been associated with complementary therapies such as acupuncture and reiki, and although HCBT doesn't necessarily fit within this camp of therapies there are some similarities; namely, the recognition that the body, mind and spirit are linked and the value of incorporating spirituality within the therapy.

In her paper on 'a mind-body-spirit' approach to treating depression and anxiety, Boynton suggests that spirituality is a missing part of therapy and she incorporates the use of yoga within standard therapy to address this gap. She describes holism, quoting Erickson's definition of holism, as follows:

> 'Holism refers to the "nature of the human being as an integral part of the universe" (Erickson, 2007). Erickson (2007) conveys that holism is a human being's natural state and any disconnection of the parts of the whole disconnects the individual from the universe. To be fully healthy is to have all aspects of body, mind, and soul intact and balanced for well-being to exist. From a holism perspective the body, mind, and spirit are completely integrated and inseparable from one another, and the parts interact dynamically and are not separate from the environment. The aim in healing is to create safety and comfort and to build or develop the resources required for the individual to reorganize the mind, body, and spirit in creating spiritual well-being. This perspective explicitly embraces the spiritual component of life in overall health and well-being.' (Boynton, 2014)

The term 'bio-psycho-social' is used fairly regularly in health care to encapsulate a holistic approach which recognises that we are social beings and that social factors shape us as well as our internal biological and psychological make up. However, we are beginning to see the term 'bio-psycho-social-spiritual' being used to acknowledge spirituality (eg. Hacker Hughes, 2017).

As you read through this book you may question the emphasis on the spiritual, but this has been to redress the balance within the CBT model. All the other aspects of the CBT model are assumed and so there is less of a focus on these because they are already standard aspects of CBT. I would like to suggest that we need to expand the model further by adding two more aspects so it becomes the 'bio-psycho-social-spiritual-cultural-environmental' model of CBT, and this is what HCBT strives to do. 'Cultural' in this model refers to any shared aspects such as beliefs, behaviours, use of language and appearance, that help to form and define a group of people such as office cultures, youth cultures as well as ethnic cultures. The environmental aspect relates to our physical environment and moves us into the areas of socio-political-economic factors such as standards of housing and employment as well as the importance of connecting with nature and recognising that we are part of a global ecosystem. With ongoing developments in internet technology and our global communication processes, we can interact with people across the world with increasing ease, which leads to the possibility of being able to see our world as one international system – an integrated whole. This was particularly evident during the Covid-19 pandemic when we shared an international fight against the virus as a world community. It is also evident with the growing response to climate change helping us to raise our awareness of our individual roles and responsibilities within a delicately balanced world-wide ecosystem.

Holism also implies bringing together diversity and the valuing of different worldviews in order to gain a broader, holistic view. This is another aspect of HCBT – drawing from psychological science as well as ancient wisdom and valuing how the diversity within these different traditions can enrich the other. It is also about valuing diversity within individuals and welcoming different viewpoints, backgrounds and life experiences within the therapy process; recognising that in sharing the parts we can better see the whole. In listening to others' perceptions of the world as a diverse group of individuals we can develop a healthier, more holistic and more accurate view of the world we share.

HCBT aims to explore different aspects of who we are in order to help people to find ways to integrate these within a balanced, healthy life. However, any model is going to fall short of fully covering all aspects of ourselves because we are such a rich mix of integrated parts in which the 'whole is far greater than the sum of the parts'. But, for now, the HCBT model has limited itself to these six main areas of our identity: the 'bio-psycho-social-spiritual-cultural-environmental' model of CBT.

Catalyst for change

Therapy is about change, and yet where does the motivation for change come from? Can people change if they have no hope that things can be different? People come to therapy because they want things to be different but some people find it hard to know what that would look like or what they really want. It is very hard to move towards something if they have never known it before or don't know what well-being looks like in their own life.

Having worked in therapy for about 30 years, I am aware that some clients come with a readiness for change and a sense of what psychologists call an 'internal locus of control' (Rotter, 1966). They believe they have some personal agency to bring about change and this makes it easier for them to engage in therapy and make progress. However, other clients come with a sense of hopelessness and apathy; they have more of an 'external locus of control': they believe that others around them have the power to make the changes needed. Often this is because they have experienced difficult childhoods or abusive relationships in which they have felt they had little choice about what they do with their lives or the day-to-day decisions they make. They may have lost touch with any sense of who they are and what they value so that their sense of self, their inner resources and true potential have been hidden away like buried treasure. They are the clients who are looking more to professionals to make change happen to them rather than creating change for themselves.

Therefore, within my own therapy practice I have found that for those most complex and traumatised clients I have needed to first focus more on what well-being could look like for them; to help them to connect with their hidden ability to make change happen. It is about first helping them to find some inner motivation or hope before they can try to make any changes happen. This involves helping people to connect with what is going well and to help them to uncover what their strengths, their values and unique potentials are as a catalyst for change, rather than just focusing on the negative and the difficulties that brought them to therapy.

A key aspect of HCBT is therefore about helping people to find their internal resources to feel that there is some possibility of change, and for them to begin to hope that things can be different for them. This involves helping people find their strengths, their interests and what naturally resonates with them – learning who they are as a unique individual that has intrinsic value and to help them to fulfil their potential.

Going beyond the standard CBT formulations

Working as a clinical psychologist and accredited CBT therapist for over 20 years, I have seen the value of CBT. I have seen how it gives people some structure to what feels like chaos in their lives, and how it offers tools to help them to begin to climb out of what seem like impossible situations. I have also used CBT on myself – challenging my own unhelpful thinking styles and setting myself goals to challenge them (such as writing this book and facing the fear of what people might think!)

However, over the years I have found myself adapting CBT in order to engage more fully with clients by incorporating what is important to them within the formulations and within the therapy. (The word 'formulation' used here simply means a summary of the different aspects in a person's development and current situation in a diagrammatic form – we will look at an example in the next chapter). This was particularly the case when I was working with clients who were experiencing psychosis (such as when people experience hearing voices and may find it difficult to think clearly, developing unusual beliefs that others see as odd or disturbing). With these individuals there were often multiple factors in their environments and life experiences that were part of our working formulation, such as violent gang experiences, racism, inadequate inner-city London housing, various faith world views and spiritual experiences and clashes of family and peer cultures leading to a confused sense of identity. These varied factors weren't often explored or even considered in the standard CBT I had been using and so I began experimenting with clients as to how we could incorporate these important factors into their personal formulations so that the client was seen more within their context than in isolation.

The majority of clients I was working with were under 30 (within Early Intervention for Psychosis services) and so there were often conversations within the therapy about identity and purpose as young people and their families grappled with the impact of psychosis. Often our later teens and 20s is the time when we focus more on our life direction and begin to ask more existential questions such as 'what is the point of life?' and 'is the path of my life something that feels a good fit with who I am?' So working with this age group for most of my NHS working life has influenced the development of HCBT and the importance of exploring identity and life's direction and purpose.

Sometimes CBT formulations can help people to see their difficulties more clearly and gives them a sense that something could change because of this awareness. However, for other clients, when they see their CBT formulations laid out before them, there can be a sense of sadness and hopelessness as they see the formulation as a map of who they are. The CBT formulation is supposed to be a diagram of their difficulty not of who they are as a whole person, and yet this can be sometimes how it is interpreted. So another aspect which started to appear in my work was drawing cycles of helpful patterns as well as maintenance cycles of unhelpful patterns and adding people's strengths as well as their difficulties.

Another strand to my therapy career was being involved in developing an IAPT service in East London. (IAPT stands for Improving Access to Psychological Therapies and was set up as a national initiative to reduce depression and anxiety in the UK, but has now broadened out to address other psychological difficulties). My experience of the early years of IAPT was that the CBT felt very manualised in comparison to my psychosis work and the contrast between these two aspects of my career helped to shape my thinking towards the formation of HCBT.

Within IAPT, I found that due to the short-term and manualised approach to CBT offered by people with a range of training and experience, there was a risk of reducing CBT to a tool box of techniques that were given out in a standardised rather than an individualised approach. The therapeutic relationship was at risk of being undervalued in short-term, guided self-help approaches. The focus was on identifying and then reducing symptoms rather than first building a therapeutic relationship within which to understand the person as a whole, within their own context. This experience helped to reinforce my thinking about the importance of understanding the individual person and their context and personalising the approach; knowing the right time to use certain CBT skills and how to adapt the CBT tools which can be used so differently for different people despite them sharing the same diagnosis.

As I began to explore these ideas in my work with clients and together, we began to develop formulations that focused more on three main areas: firstly, their sense of self or identity, and in particular their strengths; secondly, their context and the different aspects of this, and, thirdly, their spirituality. I will explore these three elements in more depth in the next chapter.

Book outline

This book is written for a wide range of people in various settings; for those interested in the theoretical concepts of HCBT as well as those who wish to use it in practice. The starting point of this book is standard CBT, and from there we explore key areas of focus that could be developed within standard CBT and which has led to the formation of the HCBT approach. The following chapters then describe the HCBT model, the developmental aspect of HCBT, and introduce the HCBT formulations. This therefore gives you the tools needed to use the HCBT approach within your own therapy practice. One key addition to standard CBT is the concept of the human spirit, which is at the heart of the HCBT model. So there is a whole chapter dedicated to exploring this concept from a wide range of sources, both spiritually and psychologically. As we move towards the end of the book we will move from theory to practice; firstly with a chapter on using the HCBT model within individual therapy and then the final chapter will show how the HCBT model is used within the Free to be Me course. This final chapter describes the HCBT process including the goals of HCBT, the group process and how the role of the group facilitator can reflect the ethos of HCBT. The book concludes with the 20 principles of HCBT as a final summary.

This book can be used on its own to develop your CBT practice or it can be used as a companion book to the Free to be Me manual, also available from Pavilion Publishing. You may find it helpful to know this theoretical background before running the Free to be Me course to get a better understanding of the ethos behind it, though I am aware that some readers may prefer to dive straight into the manual. However, I would recommend that for those wishing to run the Free to be Me course or those wishing to use the Free to be Me individual therapy approach, this book is essential reading alongside the manual.

Thank you for picking up this book and starting to read it – I hope that it is a useful tool for your own journey, whether you read it as a fellow therapist and/or as a fellow traveller on a road to wholeness for yourself.

Recommended reading as introductions to CBT

CBT was developed by Aaron Beck (1967) and this book by his daughter, Judith Beck, is a good overview of the CBT model: *Cognitive Behavior Therapy, Second Edition: Basics and Beyond*.

For a good basic introduction to CBT that is also easy to read, I would recommend the self-help book *Mind over Mood* by Dennis Greenberger and Christine Padesky.

For a more substantial text book, I would suggest *An Introduction to CBT; Skills and Applications* by David Westbrook, Helen Kennerley and Joan Kirk.

Chapter 1: A Holistic approach to CBT

Introduction

What do people want out of therapy? The common answers from clients are: to feel happy, to understand themselves and to reach various goals such as getting back to work, or having the confidence to find a new partner. Often within the NHS there is a focus on reducing symptoms – to help people be less depressed or less anxious. But there is also the aspect of self-development that is perhaps more common within the psychodynamic, existential and transpersonal forms of therapy – not just about solving problems but developing who we are as people and working towards wholeness and well-being. To borrow a quote from the Open Dialogue literature, we could also be asking 'what matters to you rather than what is the matter with you?' CBT is traditionally a problem focused approach with various CBT models having been developed to address specific mental health symptoms. However, by focusing on the problem it can sometimes be hard to visualise the solution. So by focusing on the healthy side of life and people's strengths as well as symptoms, HCBT seeks to change the perspective and focus of therapy. Helping people to identify and visualise what they are aspiring to achieve makes it easier for them to reach their goals. This idea builds on the sports psychology research which has shown that visualising and speaking about winning a race or scoring a goal increases the chance of moving towards it (eg. Vealey & Greenleaf, 2006).

HCBT seeks to be more holistic in terms of exploring self-identity and self-development as well as addressing the psychological difficulties which hinder a person reaching more of their potential. It is not just about treating the symptoms but also about developing the person. It puts the individual person at the heart of the CBT model and asks such questions as who are you, what is important to you and what do you value? The process of symptom reduction takes place in the wider context of exploring who they are and working towards meaningful goals that tap into inner strengths. It focuses on helping someone explore their unique identity and what gives them purpose and meaning in life. It then looks at the barriers both within themselves and externally that may be limiting this; hence the title of the course – 'Free to be me'. The focus is therefore as much about their potential as their symptoms.

People need a reason to change, a reason to engage with therapy and to feel that they are worth the effort. Therapy is hard work and it can be daunting to make changes and to try new things, so HCBT helps to connect people with their own inner resources that will give them the motivation and purpose to change. Becoming less depressed or less anxious happens as a by-product to this process of self-discovery through connecting with what is important to us and what is deepest within us.

CBT has developed so much over the years and has produced a wealth of models for working with different presentations such as depression, OCD, PTSD and psychosis. Standard CBT is often diagnosis based and offers a range of useful formulations adapted for these different diagnoses. In contrast, HCBT is trans-diagnostic (ie. using the same approach regardless of diagnosis or presentation) and it encourages the use of the HCBT formulation regardless of whether a person is experiencing certain mental health difficulties, has a certain diagnosis or has none. In fact, one of the main differences between HCBT and standard CBT is that HCBT has been used with people who have no diagnosable symptoms or mental health conditions, but they have attended the Free to be Me course for personal growth and greater self-awareness. So the Free to be Me course is not just for certain people who meet a criteria of diagnosis or symptoms but it recognises that we are all on a journey of personal development. This course therefore removes that division of 'healthy' and 'unhealthy' in terms of mental health and recognises that we are all on a continuum between the two, and that this is changeable. The courses that have run up to now have included people with a wide range of backgrounds, presenting difficulties and life experiences, and sometimes this range has been within the same group. This is one of the strengths of the course because it reinforces the belief that we are all working on similar things, though we may be at different stages and have different levels of functioning.

Standard CBT

To be able to use this book effectively, it is recommended that you have some knowledge already about CBT which was first developed by Aaron Beck (1967). According to the NICE (The National Institute for Health and Care Excellence) guidance for mental health, CBT is recommended for most psychological difficulties and has been shown to be an effective treatment of choice. There is a significant evidence base to support the use of CBT. For example, Butler *et al* (2006) conducted a research review of studies published between 1967 and 2004, looking at a total of 332 clinical trials with almost 10,000 participants and covering 16 diagnoses. The authors concluded that the evidence supported the efficacy of CBT across many diagnoses with particularly large effect sizes for depression, generalised anxiety disorder (GAD), panic disorder, social phobia and post-traumatic stress disorder (PTSD).

The basic premise of CBT is that our emotions, thoughts and behaviours all inter relate, and so by changing our thinking and behaviour it can help to change our emotions. In CBT we often use diagrams called formulations which help us to map out a problem and to name the factors that have contributed to the problem along with the factors that are maintaining it. A standard CBT formulation is shown in Figure 1.1: CBT Formulation.

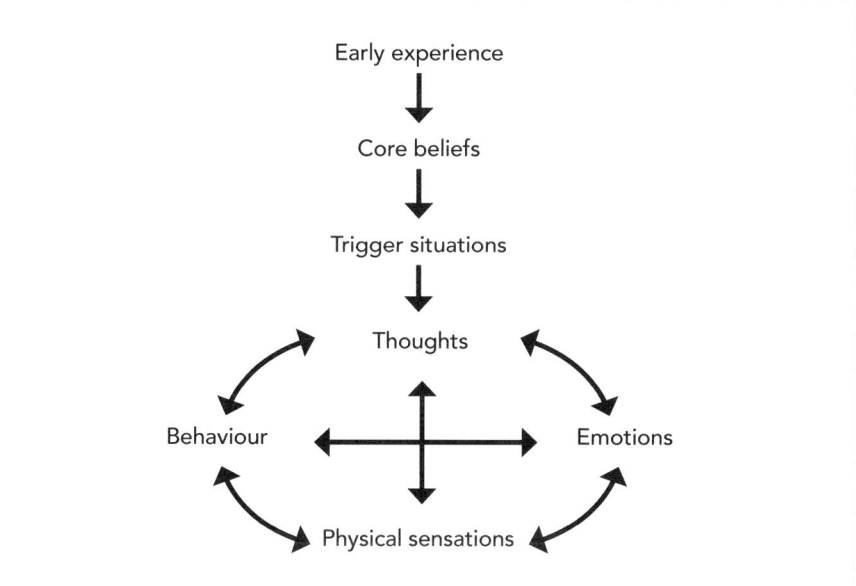

Figure 1.1: CBT formulation

For example, someone with social anxiety may have a CBT formulation like the one shown in Figure 1.2: Example of CBT Formulation. The cycle at the bottom is a key aspect of CBT and is described as the maintenance cycle – the vicious cycle that people can develop which maintains the problems they are experiencing.

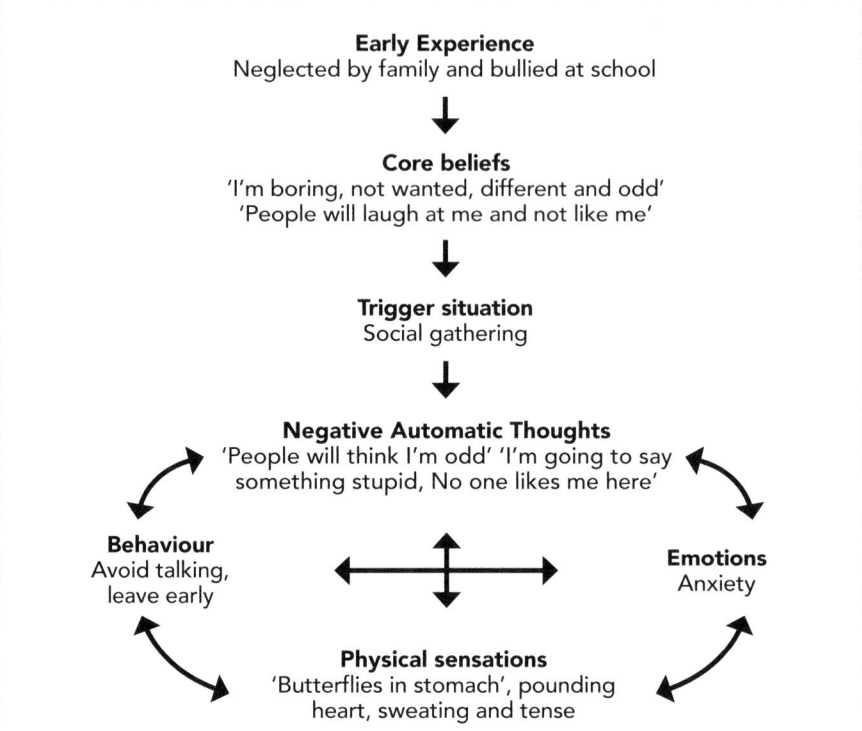

Figure 1.2: Example of CBT Formulation

CBT has different phases of therapy: firstly an assessment in which the therapist gathers all the relevant information to develop a formulation, which should be done in a collaborative way with the client so they feel it accurately reflects their problem. The next phase is the heart of the work in which various cognitive and behavioural techniques are used to help the client make changes. The final phase is bringing the therapy to an end and helping the client to become like their own therapist and to plan how they will continue the work started in therapy, once the therapy sessions have finished.

Going beyond standard CBT

If you are a mental health professional such as a psychologist or occupational therapist, or if you have run CBT groups in the past, you will be familiar with a lot of the material used within the Free to be Me course. Many of the ideas for the HCBT model and the Free to be Me course are drawn from various sources and it contains the standard CBT model. However, one of the aims of this holistic CBT model is to explicitly address those areas which are not always acknowledged, such as the importance of environmental factors on our mental health and the value of spirituality. Although some of the material may seem familiar to you, what you may find different is the focus of the course. Traditional CBT focuses on what is wrong with a person; it begins with a problem list and thinks about symptoms and what needs to change. Within HCBT the focus starts with the individual and their strengths and resources and who they are as a unique, valuable person.

Often clients in therapy say things like, 'When I become less anxious or less depressed then I will start working towards things I want to do'. In reality, we need to turn this round and help clients to see that when we start living and working towards the things we want to do, *then* we will feel less depressed or anxious instead of waiting to feel better first. This idea is seen in ACT (Harris, 2009), which encourages people to focus on values-based behaviour despite their symptoms and which we will return to towards the end of this chapter. Clients in standard CBT can focus on getting less depressed with activity diaries or work on anxiety with graded exposure but without a sense of who they are or why they are doing it, this can make it harder to be motivated to change. HCBT starts with a focus on who a person is and to help them tap into their resources and identity to fuel that drive to change. Focusing on who they are and seeing that they are worth working on gives them greater motivation to change. They may then want to reduce their depression or anxiety because they can begin to see their potential and what they have to live for.

HCBT has grown out of clinical work in response to these standard CBT formulations missing important aspects of a client's life. As part of this work, there has been a greater recognition of the important relationship between body, mind and spirit, and that improving one area can lead to improvement in the others, and the importance of assessing all three aspects. Obviously, the focus of CBT is the mind and we will explore the idea of spirit in more detail later, so at this point it is useful to highlight the importance of the body.

The body has been the traditional concern of the medical world, but the development of psychology helped to bring a balance to this biological focus by offering a window into the internal world. However, there is a danger that we can swing too far the other way, within psychology, and forget the significance of physical health and physical well-being on our mental health. This has gradually been more recognised within mental health services as a whole over recent years, with a greater emphasis on completing physical health checks, asking about basic health conditions, assessing smoking and drug and alcohol use as well as encouraging healthy lifestyles in terms of exercise, sleep and diet. It is essential to assess these areas in order to get a whole picture of a person and to clarify whether there are any physical causes to the issues for which they are seeking help.

For example, there have been examples of clients coming for therapy for panic attacks and general anxiety and an assessment of diet has shown that their daily intake is full of energy drinks, caffeine and chocolate. When changed to a more healthy diet, they experienced a decrease in their symptoms. Therapy may also explore how a person relates to and cares for their body, which is more obviously seen in body dysmorphia but can be useful to explore as part of the work around low mood, self-esteem or other issues.

Increasingly, there are examples of how working with the body can be integrated into therapy such as the use of yoga and breathing techniques as well as approaches such as dance or drama therapy. The development of body-orientated therapies has particularly grown in the field of trauma, such as Somatic Experiencing (Levine, 2010) and Sensorimotor Psychotherapy (Ogden & Fisher, 2014). Some of the ideas from these body therapies can be incorporated into standard CBT to create a more holistic approach. In particular, helping clients to identify and track physical sensations related to unhelpful or helpful cycles of thoughts, emotions and behaviours.

In terms of developing HCBT, as well as the body-mind-spirit link, there were three main areas that seemed to need a greater focus in standard CBT – firstly, the client's personal identity and in particular their strengths; secondly, their context, such as environmental and cultural influences; and thirdly their spirituality and world view. Formulations can act as road maps to direct the general direction of the therapy and ideally they need to be personalised and adapted to each individual client rather than used generically. Therefore, by just having labelled boxes for these additional areas on a formulation, this is acknowledging them in a person's life. It sends a message to the client that they can talk about these areas within therapy and that they are important areas to be explored.

Personal identity and strengths

Understanding the unique person coming into mental health services is the key basis for the therapy that will be done together. Professor Patel, former chair of the Mental Health Act Commission, described it in this way:

> 'If you don't know who I am, how are you going to provide a package of care for me to deliver something? When you do not know how important my religion is to me, what language I speak, where I am coming from, how are you going to help me cope with my mental illness? And that is what I am trying to get over to people, the first step is about identity.' (Patel, quoted in Mulholland, 2005)

Identity can include various aspects of ourselves and often therapists are familiar with the acronym social GGRRAAACCEEESSS (Burnham, 2012) to reflect on personal identity. This stands for Gender, Geography, Race, Religion, Age, Ability, Appearance, Class, Culture, Education, Ethnicity, Economics, Spirituality, Sexuality and Sexual orientation. Some of these aspects of identity may be hidden or untold and some may be visible. This model can be a useful way to explore aspects of self-identity, power and position that a person might experience relating to how they perceive themselves and how others perceive them within their context. This relates to social identity theory (Tajfel, 1979) which described how belonging to certain groups relates to a person's sense of well-being and self-esteem.

Professor Waterman, an American professor of psychology, offers this useful definition of identity which links identity with meaning and purpose:

> 'Identity refers to a person's self-definition in terms of goals, values and beliefs, whether chosen, developed through identifications or ascribed, to which there is an unwavering commitment and that therefore provides direction, purpose and meaning in life.' Waterman (2014)

The concept of identity and sense of self is often explored within CBT in terms of cognitions and in particular core beliefs about ourselves and the cognitive triad of beliefs about ourselves, the world (and in particular other people) and our future (Beck, 1976). Young (1990) developed schema therapy, in which schemas are similar to core beliefs and consist of patterns of fairly fixed views of ourselves with related behaviours, such as the schema of shame, mistrust or of failure. Both of these approaches' core beliefs tend to be centred around the negatives in a person's life, because they focus on what needs changing. So standard CBT conceptualises the individual as being made up of a combination of different levels of thoughts with a range of emotions that lead to behaviours. Together, these form consistent patterns that make up the self, which is not fixed but can be continually changing. For example, Mcleod & Ciarriochi (2012) reflect that:

> 'It would be an error to treat the self as a unitary 'thing' that is prodded and molded into better shape by CBT. Instead there are multiple aspects of self that can be described in relation to their content eg. biases in automatic attentional or memory processes for self-referent information.' (Mcleod & Ciarriochi, 2012)

Because standard CBT focuses on what is wrong with a person, the sense of self based on CBT formulations and any subsequent therapy is in danger of being negatively skewed. In reality we are an evolving, changing, rich and complex dynamic of helpful and unhelpful aspects. Depending on the context in any given situation, there will be different aspects of ourselves being expressed. So although a CBT formulation can be useful to identify key unhelpful patterns which maintain psychological difficulties, it is important that clients are not defined by these static formulations and do not view themselves predominantly in negative terms, losing sight of their strengths.

There may be some core tendencies and features which are positive, helpful qualities, as well as some unhelpful qualities within our identity. Our self isn't a solid object that we can name as 'self', but it is more like a fluid dance of familiar steps so that one individual's character can be distinguished from another. Our identities are rich and have different facets or layers – relating to different roles, relationships and settings over time. Of course, we each have some static characteristics, otherwise we wouldn't be able to recognise each other, but there is also potential for change.

Evolutionary psychologists suggest that human nature instinctively focuses on the negative rather than the positive and that we are somehow wired that way to be more alert to danger in order to survive (eg. Vaish *et al*, 2008). Often as individuals we can all too easily see what our weaknesses are and the things which we don't like about ourselves more than our strengths and our talents. Sometimes people are cautious about entering therapy because they are worried about looking too closely within themselves in case they don't like the person they find. However, despite this tendency to focus on the negative, there have been some positive developments within CBT to try to address this. For example, within Strengths-based CBT (Padesky & Mooney, 2012) virtuous cycles are drawn as well as vicious maintenance cycles in the CBT formulation, to include what is going well as well as what is unhelpful.

Positive psychology

Positive psychology has made a major contribution in highlighting what healthy well-being looks like. The leading name in this field, Martin Seligman, along with his colleagues, researched people cross-culturally and also reviewed ancient wisdom from different faith traditions, asking what makes a good life? Their work identified six core virtues: wisdom and knowledge; courage; love and humanity; justice; temperance; spirituality and transcendence. Within these virtues they identified 24 character strengths such as perseverance, hope, leadership and honesty (Seligman, 2002). Seligman initially sought to find what makes people happy but in terms of psychological health he realised that this wasn't the key question to ask, as he says:

> 'I used to think that the topic of positive psychology was happiness, that the gold standard for measuring happiness was life satisfaction, and that the goal of positive psychology was to increase life satisfaction. I now think that the topic of positive psychology is well-being and that the gold standard for measuring well-being is flourishing…' (Seligman, 2011)

Seligman and his team devised questionnaires to help people to identify their top strengths, known as their signature strengths, and found that those people who flourish are those who regularly use these. They found three common features in signature strengths, which they called the 3 Es:

- Essential – the strength feels essential to who you are as a person.
- Effortless – the strength comes without working at it and it feels natural.
- Energizing – using that strength makes you feel good and alive. (Seligman, 2002).

In order to flourish, Seligman also identified what he calls PERMA, which stands for Positive emotion, Engagement, Relationships, Meaning and Achievement (Seligman, 2011). These, he suggests, are what a person needs for well-being.

Another key concept from positive psychology is the idea of 'flow' (Csikszentmihalyi, 2008). Flow occurs when we are totally absorbed in an activity in which our strengths and skills match the challenge of the activity, leading to positive feelings of being energised. This ties in with the idea found in Eastern traditions of following 'your dharma', or purpose in life. Ancient Greeks called this eudaimonia – following your calling, which makes you feel fully alive, as compared to hedonism, which gives short-lived enjoyment and pleasure. The book *Lasting Happiness* (Parnham, 2018) develops this idea and explores how Western culture seeks health, wealth and happiness to provide contentment with life when actually, according to Parnham, what gives greater contentment is fulfilment, meaning and relationships.

Positive psychology helps people to have a more balanced, holistic view of themselves – helping people to identify their core values, character strengths and what can give them a sense of flow and their life meaning. HCBT draws from these ideas to focus more on personal strengths. The more people are able to recognise these positive aspects and find ways to develop these in their lives, the more they are going to have those positive feelings of well-being and contentment with life. So rather than focusing just on difficulties, reinforcing a person's strengths can help shift them from unhelpful maintenance cycles towards helpful cycles in which they can feel there is some positive movement towards change.

Therapy offers clinicians the privilege of hearing people's personal thoughts and struggles and we recognise that we are all very unique individuals with different potentials and strengths. Through crises and traumatic life experiences, people often discover that they are more resilient than they realised. Positive psychology has studied resilience, which has been defined as 'patterns of positive adaption during or following significant adversity' (Masten *et al*, 2009). If a material is resilient it has the ability to bounce back into shape like rubber, rather than being shattered like glass. It is often only in dire situations that we learn what an amazing resilience some people are able to discover within themselves and for them to recognise what they value in themselves and others. In positive psychology this has been encapsulated by the concept of 'post traumatic growth' (Tedeschi & Calhoun, 1995) that can develop as well as post-traumatic stress disorder (PTSD). Post traumatic growth is characterised by a fresh appreciation for life and a desire to do new things, form deeper relationships, develop spiritual growth and an awareness of our own personal strengths and abilities.

Changing language and balance of power

The language we use in talking about mental health is important in how people view themselves and how others view them too. This is especially important for those clients who feel that they have lost their sense of identity and who see themselves as defined by their symptoms. For example, if someone says '*I am* depressed' we are using the same linguistics as when we say our name or our ethnicity (such as 'I am British', 'I am Sandra'). By saying this, we are in danger of defining our inner identity as depression. Instead, by saying 'I *have* depression', we mean that the experiences that I define as depression are part of my outer expression and this is masking my inner self with its hopes and purpose, rather than defining me as a whole. How we see our mental health in relation to our identity makes a significant difference and even the suggestion that deep within us there is still hope and optimism can help someone to connect with this inner resource during periods of hopelessness and depression.

As mental health professionals, we need to avoid falling into the trap of reinforcing the idea that a person is the same as their symptoms, by working to explore different aspects of a person's identity and life and not just focusing on their difficulties and psychological problems. HCBT seeks to be aware of language and what this conveys, such as how we talk about the therapy we offer and the issues it will address. For example, from the feedback that we have received about the Free to be Me course, people have said that the title has been one of its main attractions: it has drawn people seeking to understand who they are, who is the 'real me', and to have the courage to live from that authentic place.

In the NHS we have seen the development of the recovery model, a greater focus on service user involvement and the enablement approach. These have all encouraged clients to be seen more as individuals with strengths, goals and the potential to create change and lead fulfilling lives rather than passive recipients of services from people that hold the power and who hold all the expertise. Experts by experience are now employed by many NHS trusts and are helping to slowly redress the balance of power between service users and health care professionals and to value the strengths and wisdom clients can offer that is based upon their own life experiences.

Human spirit

A basic tenet of CBT is that it is the appraisal of an event that causes distress rather than the actual event itself. So applying this to the idea of self, we can see that we can have various negative and unhelpful core beliefs about our self which differ from who we actually are, and these are unhelpful appraisals of our self. So we can have a working hypothesis about our self which can change. CBT encourages us to observe our thoughts, and by reflecting on our self clearly we can learn to recognise the unhelpful lenses we are looking through that give us a warped view of ourselves.

Some of the schemas and self perceptions are beyond a person's conscious awareness but they can still be activated. In CBT, clients are encouraged to move into the position of observer and to reflect on their negative automatic thoughts to discern if they are true or not, and also whether they are helpful or not – helpful in reaching their goals and improving their well-being.

So which part of the self is doing this deciding? Where is the bench mark for this decision of whether something is helpful or not? This is one reason that HCBT has added the concept of the human spirit into the CBT model because it helps to locate the part of us that is making this discerning decision. By adding the concept of the 'spirit' to the model, we help to identify the part of the person making that decision and that inner sense of whether something feels right or not.

Within HCBT, the spirit is seen as the deepest part of our identity. Beneath our automatic thoughts, core beliefs and emotions, it is a still centre at our heart. It is here that we can identify what resonates and rings true for us at the deepest level. The goal in HCBT is to develop a greater awareness of that inner core, the spirit, and to use it as a benchmark and resource for change. A healthy sense of self occurs when the external identity, made up of thoughts, emotions and behaviours, matches the internal self; where there is a flow of dynamic movement in response to life which is guided from the centre.

This concept of the human spirit can also be used to conceptualise our inner resources and resilience. Having listened to many stories of horrific abuse, torture and various tragedies of life, despite the evil that one person can do to another, there also seems to be something inherently good within us, our human spirit. In people's most stressful and dark times it can be this spark of life that gives them some desire to keep living and some resilience to survive. For some people this spark can be more hidden than in others, but it is still there, despite it being obscured by years of suffering or masked by the desire to cause suffering to others. Clients can be encouraged to look inwards to find this spark of life, their core identity – finding what keeps them going when they feel that life is hopeless, what they recognise as strengths within themselves, what others compliment them about, and gradually they can uncover who they are and the potential within them.

So, within HCBT the person's strengths as well as their weaknesses are explored to create a more balanced view of their identity. This at times involves a greater focus on the positives to redress our natural tendency to see the negative within ourselves. HCBT uses ideas from positive psychology and is mindful of the language used in order to reinforce a healthy sense of self. The concept of the human spirit is added to the CBT formulation to describe our inner strength and acts as a resource and inner guide for change. We will come back to this in more detail in Chapter 3.

Person in context

In CBT therapy, a person's wider context can sometimes be minimised and not discussed, and so difficulties are formulated in isolation from their social, cultural and environmental context. This can lead to a CBT formulation that suggests that a person's distress and difficulties are all down to their own unhelpful thinking. A special issue of the *Clinical Psychology Forum* (2014) highlighted this with a manifesto for social-materialist psychology. This proposed that 'distress arises from the outside inwards' and 'distress is produced by social and material influences.' (Midlands Psychology Group, 2014). In recent years, psychology has had a growing political voice in recognition that it is difficult to suggest a client makes changes in therapy while ignoring the backdrop of a life of poverty or working in unstable or unethical working conditions.

Ecological systems theory (Bronfenbrenner, 1979) can be a useful tool to keep different aspects of the environment in mind. This model is usually depicted as concentric circles around the individual beginning with the microsystem of close relationships such as family and peers and moving out to wider influences of extended family, neighbourhood to then consider the macrosystem of culture and political environments and the chronosystem which is the pattern of environmental events and changes over time. Context can involve various elements, but HCBT focuses particularly on the physical environment, the social context, and the cultural and spiritual context, by adding these to the HCBT formulation.

Environmental context

Social and environmental influences are sometimes acknowledged within CBT and are added to formulations as triggers for difficulties, for example a mother who lives in a one bedroom flat on the 13th floor with three young children is understandably more stressed than a mother living in a suburban semi with a large garden. Socio-economic factors may also be recognised as past influences in a standard CBT formulation, influencing a client's upbringing and their perception of the world. The whole field of environmental psychology shows research which supports Winston Churchill's quote in which he said: 'We shape our buildings, and afterwards our buildings shape us' (Fleury-Bahi, 2018). However, despite there being an awareness of the impact of a client's home or work environment, this may not be routinely assessed, incorporated into the formulation or considered as a possibility for change within standard CBT. Factors such as social inequality and the physical environment, despite their influence, may not be acknowledged as part of the problem, even as the backdrop to a person's formulation.

Community psychology can be helpful in exploring context, in particular by raising awareness of wider social and environmental forces. This branch of psychology is based on Lewin's theory (Lewin, 1951), which states that a person's behaviour is a function of the person, the environment and the interaction between the two. Its philosophy therefore reduces the risk of seeing a client as being responsible for their internal reactions, as if they exist in a vacuum, while ignoring the wider social and environmental forces at play. As the American community psychologist, Heller, states:

> 'We ask about queasy stomachs, sleepless nights and family conflicts but not about feeling safe in the streets, the number of persons on our block that we know by first name, or the availability of recreational centres for teens.' (Heller, 1989)

Within community psychology, there is significant research evidence to show that anxiety and aggression are:

> '…a complex result of both person and setting in combination… this has led to the adoption of ideas and terminology from ecology; for example the idea that adaption is related to the goodness of fit between person and habitat.' (Orford, 1992)

Community psychology seeks to move away from a focus on the individual and highlights the importance of social settings, systems and social power. It encourages us to look at external factors that have an impact on well-being, such as overcrowding, poor soundproofing in high-rise flats with limited outside space, levels of safety and crime rates, prejudices such as racism, socio-economic status, unemployment, and access to leisure facilities and natural spaces. Community psychology also tends to focus on prevention more than treatment, such as offering community-based awareness and well-being training or early detection of difficulties. It explores the possibility of taking psychology out into the community beyond the clinical setting. One example of this was an innovative training programme to reduce the stigma of mental health among black men in Camden, North London. This project recognised that men were more likely to open up about their difficulties to barbers. So the project trained barbers in mental health first aid, enabling them to be a link for men to get further help if needed (Camden's black barbers, 2016).

Feeling part of a community, whether that is associated to a geographical area, a virtual forum online or joining others in supporting a football team, gives us a sense of belonging and identity. As Simone Weil said in his book *The Need for Roots*:

> 'To be rooted is perhaps the most important and least recognised need of the human soul. It is one of the hardest to define. A human being has roots by virtue of his real, active and natural participation in the life of the community which preserves in living shape certain particular treasures of the past and certain particular expectations of the future.'
> (Weil, 1949)

The various long running UK soap operas portray a sense of community into which viewers can almost feel drawn as they watch. This sense of community is well reflected in the theme song from the American sitcom *Cheers*, based in a bar where, to quote the theme tune:

> 'Sometimes you want to go
> Where everybody knows your name
> And they're always glad you came
> You want to be where you can see
> The troubles are all the same…'
> (Portnoy, 1982)

Being in such a community is bound to have a positive effect on our well-being. This sense of belonging can occur even when people form a group for a particular purpose, even if it is short-term. This is part of the added benefit of group therapy where people are working through similar difficulties together as compared to individual therapy. (For example, Yalom & Leszcz, 2005) offers a good introduction to the benefits of group therapy.) This is why HCBT is ideally offered as a course rather than an individual therapeutic model because the group forms a supportive community for those who attend.

Community psychologists see the community and wider related issues as part of the problem as well as the community potentially providing the solutions. It therefore makes sense to carry out the therapy within community settings, particularly when people are reluctant to come into mental health services. In many cases psychology could be taken out of clinical settings into the communities where people live and work to make it more accessible. In developing the Free to be Me course, one of our aims was to take it beyond the statutory mental health setting and to adapt it for different cultures. For example, developing a Christian version of the course could offer some psychological input within a church context, and a Muslim version could be used in mosques and Islamic schools. By taking it to faith groups, particularly based in different ethnic cultures, HCBT could be used to reach people who may not readily seek help from mental health services. As well as being used within different faith groups, we hope to see the course taken to a wide range of community settings such as drug and alcohol services, homeless hostels and community centres. The course can then be used both as a preventative, personal development course as well as a psychological intervention.

A related area to community psychology that has become more prominent over recent years is ecotherapy, and this also has been included within the HCBT approach. As the ecotherapist Andy McGeeney says, connecting with nature improves our well-being, has no side effects, is backed by research and is free. Ecotherapy (and related fields such as wilderness therapy and green care) offers:

> '…nature-based interventions in a variety of natural settings… the common linking ethos is the contact with nature in a facilitated, structured and safe way… and is about creating a deeper connection with nature and feeling better for it.' (McGeeney, 2016)

Ecotherapy recognises that we are part of nature and as humanity has 'developed' over the centuries, the majority of the Western population has moved away from that deep interconnectedness with nature. We have lost some of that awareness that we are part of the wider ecosystem that our ancestors took for granted. Thankfully, a growing concern about climate change has helped to develop a greater awareness of our vital relationship with nature. However, the need for us to be in contact with nature as part of our well-being is still quite new within the therapeutic world. Yet we know intuitively that going out for a walk, being in beautiful countryside, stroking a pet or working on an allotment or garden can lift our spirits and help us to feel grounded and connected.

Nature encourages a transpersonal awareness of being part of something bigger than ourselves and encourages a mindful awareness and a slowing down. Nature therefore provides a therapeutic space that enables people to more readily reflect on their own internal worlds. Being in a natural environment also encourages people to reflect on their wider context and interconnection with nature. There is a rich symbolism within nature that can be brought into the therapeutic conversation such as the cycle of life seen in changing seasons and the life and death of wildlife; the sense of continuity and constancy of forests and hills; and the reliable rhythms of day following night and ocean tides. When a therapist and client are together in nature there can also be a levelling of power because the client isn't coming into the therapist's space; they are both going out together into a space which neither own nor control. It is also a space that a client can return to independently after the sessions and so this can encourage the therapeutic use of nature beyond therapy sessions.

There is a growing body of research evidence to support ecotherapy which shows that even small changes can have a major impact. For example, just putting up a picture of nature in a hospital ward can aid recovery by reducing anxiety following open heart surgery (Lunden & Ulrich, 1990). Ulrich and his colleagues also found that after as little as four minutes among trees a person's heart rate drops significantly, showing reduced stress (Ulrich *et al*, 1991). This is reflected in the ancient Japanese practice of 'forest bathing', which is the de-stressing practice of being calm and quiet, breathing deeply among trees and observing nature around you. The mental health charity MIND funded a five-year research programme called Ecominds, made up of 130 ecotherapy projects. Their findings showed that 70% of participants had a significant improvement in their mental well-being and measures of self-esteem increased for two thirds of participants. They also found improvements in social involvement, with participants getting more involved in community activities after the project as a result of being part of an ecotherapy group. There was also a rise in participants having an ongoing connection with nature and improved environmentally friendly practices beyond the ecotherapy (Bragg *et al*, 2013). Biophilia is the concept that people have an inherent affinity for nature and this has led to an area of architecture called biophilic design. This recognises the importance of connecting with nature and promotes building designs which have a greater connection with nature in order to improve well-being (Kellert, 2018).

Social context

So far we have explored the environmental context of a person, highlighting the importance of socio-economic factors, the community and a person's connection with nature. Now we will consider a person's social context.

We are, to some degree, the people we are because of the relationships we have experienced. People we spend time with shape us and influence us, as do the authors we read, who we follow on social media and who we watch on TV. The most rewarding and most painful moments of our lives are often related to relationships. In psychology we have benefited from the systemic schools of therapy which formulate problems as being due to difficulties within relationships. Systemic therapy sees people as part of a network or 'system' of people that all interact and influence each other. They have taught us that problems are located within these systems of relationships, such as a family, as well as internally within a person. Family therapy therefore helps to change distress by changing the system and the family dynamics.

The system is also part of the solution and there is significant research confirming that it is the support from those around us that is often what helps us to get through difficult life experiences:

> 'The breadth and consistency of the research and the beneficial effects of social support are impressive… Either through direct protective effects or by buffering the adverse consequences of life stress, social support is associated with a decreased likelihood of developing disorder.' (Munroe & Steiner, 1986)

There are some helpful models within this systemic literature that can be incorporated to develop a more systemic view within CBT such as the use of genograms (similar to family trees) and the 'co-ordinated management of meaning' model (Pearce, 1976). This model describes the different levels of influence on a person, consisting of cultural beliefs, family stories, beliefs within relationships and individual beliefs and how these influence the meaning we give to communication. Some attempts have been made to incorporate systemic views into CBT, particularly in children and adolescent mental health services. For example, Dummett (2006) developed a systemic cognitive-behavioural therapy model for working with children and families which incorporated developmental, attachment, family and systemic influences.

CBT often explores a client's relationship dynamics and the effect their relationships have on them. However, this is not always added to the standard CBT formulation unless it is identified as a trigger or a past influence. Similarly, CBT has sometimes involved teaching social skills when needed, such as assertiveness training and helping people to improve their social connections, but again this is not always routine practice. The area of relationships has therefore been a focus which HCBT has wanted to develop further.

CBT is quite an individualistic approach and so it is in danger of inferring that a client is totally at fault for their psychological difficulties; that it is due to their unhelpful thinking and responses to a situation. This is part of our wider Western culture of individualism that has been described as 'liquid modernity' by sociologist Zygmunt Bauman:

> 'individualized, privatised version of modernity leaves the burden of pattern-weaving and the responsibility for failure falling primarily on the individual's shoulders.' (Bauman, 2000)

Standard CBT focuses on helping people recognise their unhelpful thoughts and this can sometimes lead to clients blaming themselves and feeling fully responsible for how they think. Recognising the wider social context within CBT can potentially help to reduce this sense of blame that some clients can feel, recognising that their responses are understandable within the contexts in which they live.

Western society is typically individualistic and therefore the individualistic style of CBT may suit clients from this background. However, greater emphasis on social systems may help to engage clients from other cultures where the extended family plays a greater role and where the world view is less individualistic than in Western cultures. For some cultures, there cannot be a sense of wholeness and personal growth if it is not shared with others within their family and social network. So a therapy which emphasises the value of healthy relationships is important for all cultures but particularly for those that are more community based. Peter Gilbert, a senior social worker, reflected on personal well-being as being dependent on the good of all, stating:

> 'Aristotle, as we know, did not speak of "happiness" as an individualistic concept, but about "flourishing" as a way of aligning the personal with the civic, rights with responsibilities, personal enjoyment with altruism. The enlightenment thinkers, Rousseau, Diderot, Montesquieu and others, also saw that individuality and liberty had to be placed in a social context.' (Gilbert, 2011)

One example of this importance of community is the South African concept of Ubuntu, which was described by Bishop Desmond Tutu in this way:

> '…a person is a person through other persons, that my humanity is caught up, bound up, inextricably, with yours.' (Tutu, 2008)

Ubuntu is described as mutual recognition and respect which leads to mutual care and sharing so that those in the community are available to others and are not threatened by other people's success or ability. This means that life is built on co-operation rather than competition. Within this concept is the understanding that a person cannot be well if those around them, including the well-being of their natural environment, do not share their personal well-being.

Cultural and spiritual context

Culture is another key context for a person, and yet cultural influences are not routinely added to standard CBT formulations. Often when we think of culture, we tend to think of ethnicity, but there are also many non-ethnic cultures: youth cultures, gaming cultures or office cultures. Different organisations and workplaces create their own cultures, such as the culture within the NHS. These different cultures can have a significant impact on well-being and can influence a person's internal sense of self and identity. Although work, culture and social groups may be recognised within standard CBT, they may not be added within a standard CBT formulation and so not explored in detail.

HCBT therefore seeks to give these cultural issues a greater focus. The 'Black Lives Matter' movement is a powerful reminder of the need to see the cultural context of a person and to understand how issues such as institutional racism can impact on personal well-being. The Black Lives Matter movement also acts as a powerful example of how people standing together with a shared world view can empower individuals and so improve self-esteem and a healthier sense of self.

The importance of ethnic culture within CBT has been the focus of a growing body of research showing that CBT can be adapted for different cultures. For example, Naeem *et al* (2010) adapted CBT for South Asian Muslims, and Propst *et al* (1992) adapted CBT for American Christians. Rathod *et al* (2010) carried out a qualitative study to explore how mental disorders were perceived by different cultures through interviewing service users, health care professionals and members of different cultural communities. The study focused on four cultural communities – Afro-Caribbean, Black African, Bangladeshi and Pakistani. They found that the top two explanations for mental illness within these communities were that mental ill health was due to previous wrong doing or had a supernatural explanation, such as due to jinn or an evil spirit. (Within Islam, jinn are seen as created beings that are different to humans and other spiritual beings.) Service users with these beliefs are therefore more likely to visit a traditional healer, the priest, Imam or other source of religious support, rather than seeking help from mental health services. The researchers went on to develop a culturally adapted form of CBT which incorporated these different world views (Rathod *et al*, 2010). Within psychology along with other academic fields there is a growing awareness of how Eurocentric views have dominated many areas of study and that different cultural and spiritual viewpoints, such as African centred views or black psychology, can be used to bring a more holistic approach, particularly when working with clients from different cultural backgrounds (eg. McInnis, 2017).

The HCBT model sees a person in context and identifies the different external influences on that person. As we can see from the research by Rathod and his colleagues, this can involve beliefs about spiritual influences. Most of the world's faith traditions have beliefs about a spiritual world that has an influence on the physical world we can see. This might include beliefs in a god, angels, evil spirits or other supernatural beings that can interact with a person in some way. These external spiritual influences can be a significant part of a client's understanding of their mental well-being and if these are ignored then this will limit the shared understanding between client and therapist, and a client may disengage from therapy. So HCBT acknowledges spiritual influences within the model, if this is in line with the client's belief system. For example, a belief that is sometimes seen amongst Muslims who are experiencing psychotic symptoms is the belief that jinn are responsible. A formulation which acknowledges and includes this belief will help to develop a shared view of the difficulties and also encourages a mutual agreement of possible treatment options such as prayer and reading the Quran, alongside traditional CBT and medication. Including spiritual influences in a formulation gives the client an invitation to share their spiritual beliefs and these can then be incorporated into the formulation alongside psychological explanations. This leads to a 'both/and' approach to the spiritual and psychological, rather than getting into the difficult conversations of an 'either/or' approach. Despite the clinician's personal views on spiritual influences, this approach can lead to a greater understanding of different views and a more collaboratively agreed formulation as a basis for therapy.

So, within HCBT the different aspects of a person's context are explored, and in particular the environmental, social, cultural and spiritual influences.

Personal spirituality

A report by the Department of Health reviewing the role of religion in health care, stated that:

> '…an holistic approach to the patient, which takes account of their physical, cultural, social, mental and spiritual needs would seem to have a particular significance within mental health services. Spirituality and an individual's religion or beliefs are increasingly acknowledged as playing an important role in the overall healing process.' (Department of Health, 2009)

Defining spirituality

We have already mentioned the idea that spiritual influences are part of a person's wider context, but now we will focus on the idea of spirituality as a more general term.

Spirituality is not synonymous with religion and faith. Rather it relates to how an individual seeks to answer existential questions such as 'who am I?' and 'why am I here?' It is about having a framework that gives a sense of purpose and meaning to life as well as a sense of belonging to something bigger than themselves. This may be through a faith but may equally be through other avenues such as connecting with nature, creating music and art or serving the community in some way.

The Bradford District Care NHS Foundation Trust describes spirituality in their Spiritual well-being policy as being:

> '…the essence of human beings as unique individuals "What makes me, me and you, you?" So it is the power, energy and hopefulness in a person. It is life at its best, growth and creativity, freedom and love. It is what is deepest in us – what gives us direction, motivation. It is what enables a person to survive bad times, to be strong, to overcome difficulties and to become themselves.' (Bradford District Care, 2001)

William Bloom, who describes himself as a modern Western mystic, describes it in this way:

> 'Spirituality is everybody's natural connection with the wonder and energy of life and the instinct to explore and understand it – connect, reflect and serve.' (Bloom, 2019)

For some people, spirituality is expressed through their faith and being part of a religion. A religion can be defined as a structure in which people share a specific spirituality which usually focuses on a belief in a god or spiritual being, and they have shared beliefs, styles of worship, holy books and a faith tradition. So, for those in a faith tradition, one way of seeing the difference between religion and spirituality is that the former are shared practices and beliefs whereas the latter is about an individual's journey and experiences in personalising these shared externals of their religion.

Although numbers of people affiliated to religions is in decline in the West, there is a growing group of people who identify as 'Spiritual But Not Religious' and people seem to be interested in developing a more individualised spirituality (Christopherson, 2020). There has also been an ongoing number of people having spiritual experiences regardless of faith or cultural background. In 1969, Sir Alister Hardy started the Religious Experience Research Centre at Oxford University to collect first-hand experiences of people from across the world who had had a spiritual or religious experience. The centre continues to collect these and has an archive of over 6,000 accounts of different spiritual experiences (Hardy, 1979).

The value of incorporating spirituality in therapy

Considering the above definitions of spirituality, it seems that because spirituality can be a resource of 'power, energy and hopefulness' then it would be useful to harness within therapy. A person's spirituality could potentially be a valuable motivator towards change if it was accessed and explored as part of the process of change. The research on spirituality seems to support this and has shown that spirituality can be a significant source of purpose and strength for many people. For example, Dein (2010) reviewed the literature on spirituality and mental health and concluded that 'patients with psychiatric disorders frequently use religion to cope with distress'. Another review of 3,300 studies conducted between 1872 and 2010 concluded that spirituality or religious affiliation can lead to better mental health and well-being, reduced stress, an increase in positive emotions, giving meaning to adversity and enhancing one's sense of purpose and increased adaptability to problems (Koenig *et al*, 2012).

The Royal College of Psychiatrists, in their booklet on spirituality and mental health, states:

> 'Spirituality involves a dimension of human experiences that psychiatrists are increasingly interested in, because of its potential benefits for mental health… evidence for the benefits for mental health of belonging to a faith community, holding religious or spiritual beliefs, and engaging in associated practices, is now substantial.' (RCP, 2006)

In seeking to understand why spirituality may be of benefit, James and Wells (2003) suggested that spirituality has a positive effect on mental health by providing helpful cognitive-behavioural mechanisms such as self-regulation of thinking processes and a cognitive framework by which people appraise life events in a healthy way. For a significant number of service users, their faith is central to their life and has a key role to play in how they understand and manage their mental well-being and yet often it is not discussed within therapy (Koenig *et al*, 2012).

Although spirituality can be a great source of support, it is also important to highlight that some aspects of religion can also reinforce psychological difficulties if it involves unhelpful beliefs and behaviours. In the same way that there may be aspects of a client's family that can be helpful and unhelpful, and this is explored through the therapy process, a person's spirituality may be explored in a similar way. For example, the American psychologist Kenneth Pargament researched different religious coping strategies and found that religious beliefs that encouraged passive ways of coping, such as 'God will sort it all out', were associated with poorer mental health compared to more proactive, helpful ways of coping, such as 'God and I will work this out together' (Pergament *et al*, 1998). People may also have unhealthy views of a god who is harsh and punishing, which could reinforce their sense of low self-worth. Spirituality can therefore be part of the solution or part of the problem, or a combination of both, and so by ignoring this area it could limit the assessment of the whole person. By including spirituality into therapy, we can begin to recognise any unhelpful factors that may undermine the therapy process and also help to identify positive resources that could be used within the therapeutic process such as a person's values and motivation for change.

Spirituality within CBT

This research would therefore suggest that incorporating spirituality into the therapy process would be helpful. Although not addressed explicitly, spiritual beliefs are sometimes explored in CBT through identifying thoughts and behaviours from a person's spirituality. There have been a number of suggestions as to how spirituality can be incorporated into CBT, but these have predominantly focused on incorporating specific religious beliefs within CBT rather than spirituality in general. For example, CBT has been adapted for Christianity (eg. Propst *et al*, 1992), for Judaism (eg. Paradis *et al*, 1996) for Islam (eg. Azhar & Varma, 2000) and for Taoism (Zhang *et al*, 2002). A literature review by Hodge on different forms of spiritually modified cognitive therapy reviewed 14 studies in which the client's spiritual worldview was incorporated into therapy and clients showed improvements in their mental health similar to those seen in standard treatment (Hodge, 2006). There is also evidence that clients with a faith prefer working with therapists who recognise the importance of that faith and who integrate it into therapy (eg. Post & Wade, 2009) and that therapy is more effective if it integrates a client's religious beliefs (eg. Propst *et al*, 1992).

There have been a few adaptations to CBT to incorporate spirituality in general, rather than adapting CBT to include aspects of a particular faith tradition. One example of incorporating spiritualty in CBT is described by Hodge (2008) who offers a generic 'Spiritually modified CBT'. In this model he rephrases CBT principles using clients' spiritual terminology and beliefs in order to develop spiritually based self-statements in changing unhelpful thoughts for religious clients. Dr D'Souza, a consultant psychiatrist in Australia, along with his colleagues developed 'Spiritually augmented cognitive behaviour therapy' (SACBT), and they defined spirituality as:

> 'the ways in which people fulfil what they hold to be the purpose of their lives. Spirituality can encompass belief in a higher being, the search for meaning and a sense of purpose and connectedness.' (D'Souza *et al*, 2002)

Their Spiritually augmented CBT incorporates existential ideas in order to help clients to find meaning and to validate and incorporate their spiritual beliefs and practices into individual therapy. Their randomised control trial showed significant improvements compared to supportive counselling and also showed that clients were more likely to stay in this therapy compared to standard CBT (D'Souza *et al*, 2002). Rob Waller *et al* (2010) also suggested a model that incorporates spirituality in general, rather than incorporating a particular faith tradition. They suggested seven key principles to help therapists incorporate spirituality into CBT and also proposed a three-domain model of behavioural, cognitive and existential domains with the later one addressing spirituality.

In 2005, the relationship between CBT and spirituality was explored in a conversation between the founder of CBT, Aaron Beck, and the 14th Dalai Lama at the International Congress of Cognitive Psychotherapy in Göteborg, Sweden. Aaron Beck and the Dalai Lama discussed areas of overlap between CBT and the spirituality of Buddhism. Their conversation reflected on how negative thoughts and emotions are often grounded in self-centeredness and how egocentricity could lead to unhappiness by making people feel isolated and inwardly focused on their negative emotions. They suggested that, as people learn to see life from a more holistic perspective and feel as if they are part of the larger human network, then distress is more easily managed. This is because they are connecting with something greater than themselves and are more outward looking. Within the conversation, there was a recognition that spirituality could help to bring this healthier focus (Mind over Mood, 2012).

Improving engagement

Mental health services, particularly in urban settings, are accessed by service users who come from a wide range of cultural and spiritual backgrounds. Therapists therefore need to be aware of their service users' world views and in particular how they understand mental health. Although the evidence to support the use of CBT is strong, if clients see this approach as irrelevant to their world view and to their understanding of mental health, then engagement with services could be hindered. For example, the work done by Rathod *et al* (2010), which was referred to earlier in this chapter, highlighted how people with spiritual views are more likely to seek help from their own religious communities instead of mental health services. This is partly because they know that the person they are talking to shares the same world view as them, but also because they perceive the mental health services as, at best, uninterested in the spiritual and at worst pathologising the spiritual (Dein *et al*, 2010). This suggests that a therapy such as HCBT, which allows space to explore spirituality, would help clients for whom spirituality is an integral part of their life, to feel that the therapy is addressing them as a whole person. It would offer a useful approach in helping clients with different spiritual views to engage with mental health services. This is particularly important to recognise because mental health services tend to be seen as secular environments where spiritual issues are not considered (Dein *et al*, 2010). For example, there is a recognised 'religiosity gap' between mental health professionals and service users, with psychiatrists – and in particular psychologists – being less religious than service users (Frazier & Hansen, 2009). If a client raises a spiritual issue within therapy it is sometimes seen as a separate issue that needs addressing by a chaplain or another service rather than something that could be explored within therapy. Following a national survey of psychotherapists in the US, Bergin and Jensen concluded that:

> 'Secular approaches to psychotherapy may provide an alien values framework … a majority of the population probably prefers an orientation to a spiritual perspective. We need to better perceive and respond to this public need.' (Bergin & Jensen, 1990).

If people of faith seek help within a religious setting there is the risk of their difficulty being seen solely as a spiritual problem, and this could lead to a situation in which the client could be reluctant to seek professional help or take psychiatric medication. Equally, if the spiritual is ignored within health services, the treatment fails to be truly holistic and the client may disengage. CBT is therefore likely to engage clients better and be more effective if the shared formulation and therapeutic approach integrates a client's world view and spiritual beliefs within the CBT and addresses the spiritual, psychological and physical aspects. This is one reason why the Free to be Me course was developed to include the spiritual and why it is also being adapted into Christian and Muslim versions to be used in faith community settings.

Therefore, to gain a deeper understanding of the individual, it seems appropriate to incorporate a person's spirituality into CBT and to understand how this interacts with the difficulties they wish to address.

What would an holistic approach add to CBT?

So HCBT seeks to develop standard CBT by focusing more on a person's identity and strengths; exploring the external context of the person, namely their environment, culture and social and spiritual influences and also to focus more on their spirituality. Other developments of CBT have also sought to broaden standard CBT and these are collectively known as contextual or third wave CBT approaches, which includes ACT (Acceptance and Commitment Therapy), DBT (Dialectical Behaviour Therapy), Mindfulness CBT and Compassion Focused therapy.

As well as looking at the content of thoughts, third wave CBT explores the relationship we have with these thoughts, for example whether we choose to focus on them or not or being able to let our thoughts pass without getting emotionally entangled by them. Third wave approaches have introduced mindfulness to CBT which has been a significant step in broadening the CBT approach, and we will return to third wave CBT approaches when we look at the concept of the human spirit in Chapter 3.

Standard CBT tends to divide a person into their different psychological aspects such as thoughts, emotions and behaviour. This is useful to help us to understand how these aspects interact and to determine what can be focused on to create change. However, there is also the need to look at the whole picture – to see that the whole is greater than the sum of the parts and also to explore what that 'whole' looks like. As the analytical psychotherapist Carl Jung said:

> 'The continuity of nature knows nothing of those antithetical distinctions which the human intellect is forced to set up as helps to understanding. The distinction between mind and body is an artificial dichotomy … so intimate the intermingling of bodily and psychic traits… If I recognise

> only naturalistic values and explain everything in physical terms, I
> shall depreciate, hinder or even destroy the spiritual development of
> my patients. And if I hold exclusively to a spiritual interpretation, then
> I shall misunderstand and do violence to the natural man in his right
> to existence as a physical being … there is a need to recognise both as
> constituent elements of one psyche.' (Jung, 1933)

CBT is a valuable therapy model that highlights the interaction between various parts of the maintenance cycles within formulations, but there is also a need to then stand back and look at the person as a whole. In particular, not just their difficulties and unhelpful patterns of thoughts and behaviour but to reflect on their strengths, their potential and to also see helpful cycles and patterns.

So, to conclude this introduction, why has HCBT been developed? It has been developed in response to aspects of life which clients have brought into the therapy room and are in danger of being side-lined within standard CBT. Standard, and in particular short-term manualised CBT, carries the risk of reinforcing a client's attention on symptoms without really asking more about who the client is as a person and tapping into their strengths and what motivates them to change. In some ways this could be as simple as a change in our language and a greater focus within existing therapy on individual strengths and hopes. It could also involve a shift to increasing the positives instead of decreasing the negatives, such as reinforcing personal talents and meaningful activities rather than just working on reducing symptoms of depression or stress. If someone comes to therapy saying they want to be less depressed but they are sitting at home, isolated from the world watching TV most of their day, is an hour of CBT to change some of their negative thoughts or start some behavioural activation, really going to change their world? Don't we also need to explore their wider context and the impact of this on any goals, to understand their values and to help them to find a purpose in life and a way of connecting with others? Thankfully, much of CBT that is offered does explore these issues and many people also have enough motivation and inner resources to use CBT to make significant changes. However, some clients need more support to explore these wider issues and to begin to connect with their strengths and see their potential.

HCBT has been developed to address some of these gaps in CBT; to focus more on their individuality with their own uniqueness and strengths; to see a person more in their context and to consider the impact of this context; and thirdly to incorporate spirituality into CBT. HCBT seeks to recognise that there are many factors that need to be considered if we are going to see the person as a whole being, and all these factors inter-relate. So, to return to the Open Dialogue question from the beginning of the chapter, it is about moving from 'What's the matter with you?' to 'What matters to you?' By asking these sorts of questions we begin to understand what can bring change. The person first needs to find a reason to change. They need to begin to believe that they are worth changing, that their life can have some purpose and that they have some value as an individual. They need to know that if they do make changes then there is the possibility of finding a meaningful life waiting for them that only they can live and is based on who they are. This is what is at the heart of HCBT.

Chapter 2: The holistic CBT model

Developing a holistic approach

There are various forms of therapy and mental health support available. If we were to caricature it a little, we could imagine someone – let's call them Joe – coming to therapy because he is depressed. Depending on what type of therapist he sees, each would have a different focus and a different explanation of why Joe is depressed, similar to those shown in Figure 2.1: Different perspectives in therapy

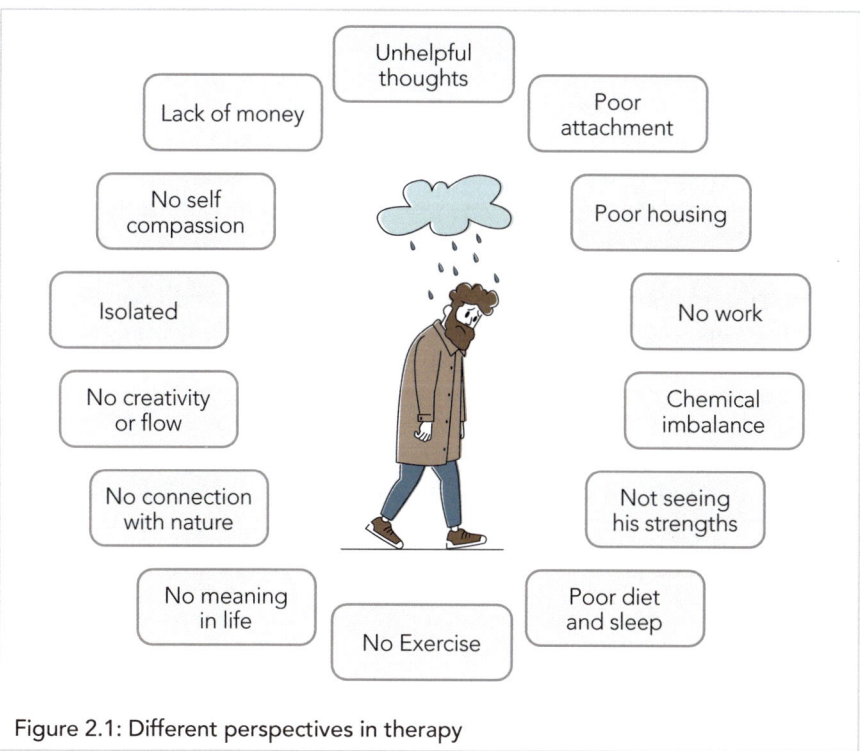

Figure 2.1: Different perspectives in therapy

This is obviously a caricature of therapies as most therapists and health care workers would cover a number of these factors and would aim to work in a holistic manner. However, to borrow a phrase, if we are trained to be a hammer then there is a danger of seeing everyone as a nail. Each therapist and mental health professional is trained to look at a person through a certain lens. For example, a doctor focuses on diagnoses and offers psychiatric medication where as a systemic therapist will be focusing on relationships within the social network. We can address psychological difficulties and personal development in so many different ways. Therefore a holistic model is in danger of just getting bigger and bigger and more cumbersome. By focusing on so many factors it can become difficult to keep the whole person in mind. This is why, ideally, mental health teams are made up of different professions working alongside the client and their support network to develop a multidimensional care plan centred round the client. By having a multi-professional team, the different health care professionals can keep different aspects of the client in mind to develop a shared formulation through their various viewpoints. The challenge in creating a truly holistic therapy is to hold each of these different areas of focus in balance while trying to hold the whole person in mind.

Holistic therapeutic approaches

There have been a range of developments within psychology over the years designed to create more holistic approaches to therapy. One of the first holistic approaches was Lazarus' multimodel therapy (Lazarus, 1976). This used the acronym BASIC ID to highlight the areas which need addressing in therapy and stands for Behaviour, Affect, Sensation, Imagery, Cognition, Interpersonal relationships, and Drugs/Biological processes. (If he had added the spiritual it could have become BASIC SID!)

One of the first holistic approaches to integrate spirituality in therapy was Psychosynthesis (Assagioli, 1965). This sought to combine spirituality and psychology in order to help people learn more about themselves and become more integrated. This integration of spirituality and psychology falls under the umbrella of transpersonal psychology. One of the key figures in this field is Ken Wilber with his work on integral psychology (which we will briefly explore later). Other examples of therapies which seek to bring spirituality into psychology are psycho-spiritual integrative therapy (Garlick *et al*, 2011) and the spiritual self-schema development programme (Avants & Margolin, 2004). As we saw in Chapter 1, along with some of the third wave CBT approaches, there are various CBT approaches that have added a spiritual element such as spiritually augmented CBT and other culturally and religiously adapted CBT approaches.

Along with a growing body of research and practice within transpersonal psychology, there has also been the growing area of holistic psychology. This field of psychology offers therapy that recognises the relationship between body, mind and spirit by integrating practices such as body work, yoga, breathing techniques, creativity, nutrition, spirituality and other complementary and holistic practices.

In terms of being more holistic, we could also consider the balance between the right and left hemispheres of the brain, highlighted in Iain

McGilchrist's book *The Master and His Emissary* (McGilchrist, 2009). The thesis of his book challenges us to consider how much therapy, and particularly CBT, is biased towards the more mechanical and compartmentalising functions of the brain. His work encourages the use of symbols and images as well as words and so supports the idea of integrating creative therapies within CBT.

Identity formation

Before introducing the HCBT model, it is useful to pause first to consider how we view identity formation in order to understand the role of spirit within this model. The psychologist Alan Waterman, in considering how our identity develops, offers some useful ideas in comparing two main perspectives. The first is the existential approach of how our identity is formed suggested by philosophers such as Jean-Paul Sartre, in which we create our identities by the choices we make. In this process we have total freedom to choose who we become and also have total responsibility for our identity. In existentialism there is the potential that our identity could be forever adapting, depending on what we choose. Waterman compares this existential thinking to the ideas of the psychiatrist Victor Frankl, who developed logotherapy, and which he labels as essentialism. This approach suggests that we have certain inbuilt tendencies and attributes which are more fixed, similar to our genetic make up. Essentialism suggests that each person has some sort of existing essence which needs to be uncovered and developed. Waterman concludes that in reality our identity is formed through a combination of existentialism and essentialism; we each have some sort of true nature or essence which we can then develop or shape according to our free choices and the directions we take in life (Waterman, 2014).

The HCBT approach is based on this idea of a combination of both essentialism and existentialism. The concept of the spirit within the HCBT model represents this form of essence or true nature and is seen to be a relatively stable core aspect of our identity. It represents our potential and the source of our inner strength and wisdom. However, there is also the aspect of existentialism where the choices we make either move us towards well-being and growth or away from this. Through various life choices, we can develop a range of created identities to portray ourselves in a certain light in order to fit in with peers or to succeed in certain roles. Our spirit or essence can therefore be hidden by layers of created identities or our spirit may be more visible as an authentic identity, depending on the choices we make.

HCBT adapts the CBT idea of helpful and unhelpful cycles and explores the idea that, simplistically speaking, people make helpful choices which can uncover and develop this essence, or unhelpful choices that bury it deeper. The more a person develops and lives from their essence or spirit and their outer identity is in line with their spirit, then the more they develop into a healthier version of themselves as a whole being. On the other hand, the more they live out of identities which do not resonate with their inner spirit then the more they develop an unhealthier version of themselves. We will return to this more developmental aspect of HCBT in Chapter 4 but for now let's focus on the basic HCBT model.

HCBT model

As we explored in the previous chapter, HCBT seeks to be more holistic than standard CBT by adding a greater focus on identity, personal strengths, context and spirituality. At the heart of the HCBT model is the added concept of the spirit which helps us to consider these different aspects within CBT and we will explore this concept further in the next chapter. The challenge is that the more holistic we try and make our model of therapy, the more complicated and complex it becomes. However, at the same time we need a basic model and formulation which is not too complicated and is a useful map for the therapy.

This model can be likened to following the London tube map which, as someone else has once said, cannot fully reflect the rich experience of travelling round London but can act as a useful guide for us to make the journey. There is a dilemma of wanting to keep the big picture in mind, of seeing a whole person in their whole context, and yet also dividing the person into boxes in order to ensure that we are not forgetting key aspects whilst capturing that big picture.

The HCBT model is pictured in a diagrammatical way in Figure 2.2: The HCBT model. It separates the psychological (thoughts and emotions), physical and spiritual parts of an individual and also introduces the contextual influences. This acts as a framework to explore who we are as unique individuals.

Internal aspects

The outer circle is the body, the physical structure of the person through which a person receives incoming information via their senses. This information is processed by their brain and nervous system which leads to internal responses. In standard CBT we are already familiar with these internal responses of thoughts and emotions leading to behaviours carried out through the body. The focus of this circle is on behaviour and physiological responses which are important factors in standard CBT. However, adding the body to a CBT model in this way highlights the importance of the body and its interaction with psychological well-being. This interaction is sometimes addressed in standard CBT therapy by encouraging a healthy lifestyle with a balanced diet and regular exercise, but this is not always an intrinsic part of the CBT model. The interaction between the body and the psychological well-being of a person may only be addressed in traditional CBT when significant difficulties are recognised in this area. However, the HCBT model encourages a more routine approach to focusing on the body and on the interaction between the physical, psychological and spiritual.

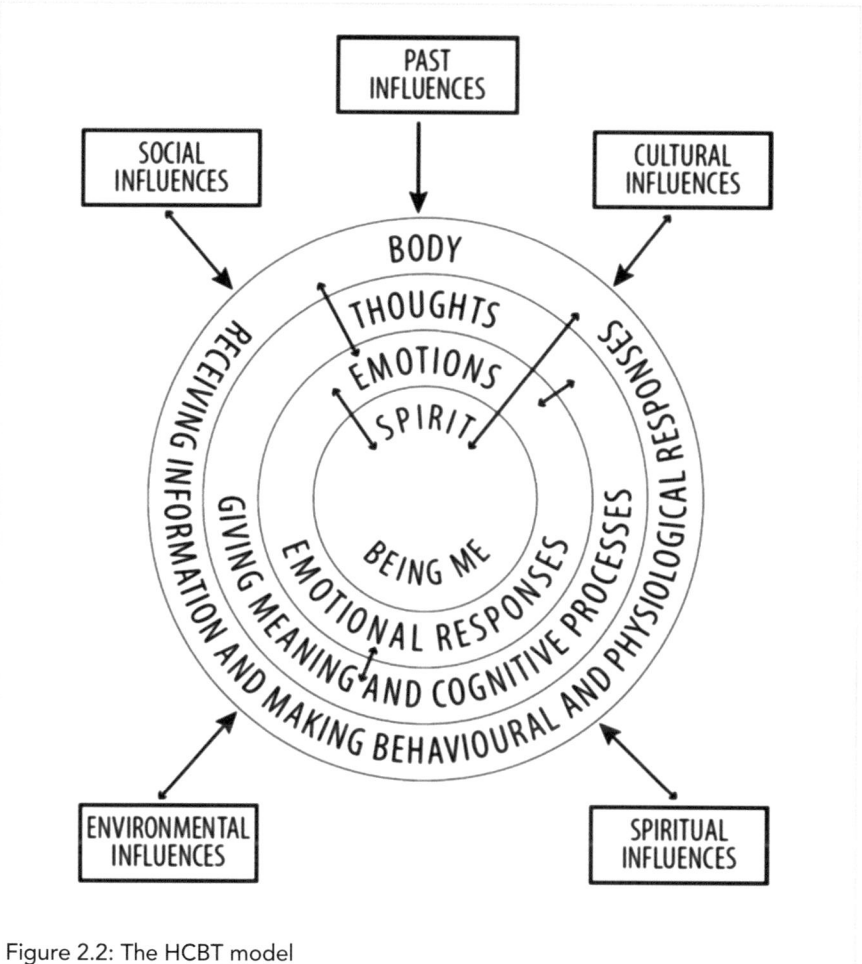

Figure 2.2: The HCBT model

The next circle represents thoughts which, as in standard CBT, give meaning to the information received by the body. The circle of thoughts includes three different aspects of cognitive function – firstly the content of thought, that is, what we actually think such as, 'it's going to rain today'; secondly, cognitive processes such as attention, for example ruminating on the fact that it's raining more than focusing on the forecast for sun later; thirdly, there are metacognitive thoughts (thoughts about thoughts) such as 'I'm such a pessimist for focusing on this rain'. As external information is received and processed by the body this leads to cognitive appraisals so that the information is given meaning by the person. As in standard CBT, there are different layers of thoughts such as core beliefs, underlying assumptions (sometimes called 'rules for living') and automatic thoughts. The automatic thoughts can be rooted in persistent core beliefs or cognitive biases which the person has developed.

The third circle represents the emotions that are produced as a response to thoughts and are experienced physiologically in the body. Both internal and external experiences are cognitively appraised and physiological sensations are named based on these appraisals. For example, the physical sensation of anxiety is much the same as excitement – feeling flushed, short of breath and racing heart. Our mind translates these physiological reactions according to the data it is gathering from the context and from past experiences. The collected data is used to make a decision as to whether the physiological sensations can be labelled as excitement or anxiety, or possibly a bit of both. Emotions may also result from a direct physiological reflex response from the body such as the 'fight, flight, freeze' response. Together these two circles of thoughts and emotions are the psychological aspect of the person, and over time they form our characteristics and identities, and so along with our physical self, they form external versions of ourselves.

Up to this point this model is very similar to standard CBT, but HCBT adds another key component. At the centre is the spirit of the person which, as has already been discussed, is the core of a person that is unique to them. The term 'spirit' will be defined differently by different clients and so the HCBT model acknowledges this and does not define the term too rigidly. They may also choose a different word which is more aligned to their worldview such as 'heart', 'identity' or 'consciousness', as we will explore further in the next chapter.

The arrows going between each of the circles are not meant to be exhaustive but are to illustrate that the different sections interact in a constant exchange between these different aspects of a person. A holistic approach to therapy encourages an ongoing awareness of the person as a whole and that there are constant interactions between these different levels. Information can be received at each section and responses can be made at each section and each section influences the others. For example, thoughts and feelings may result from external influences or maybe from a person's spirit within them. The cognitive models of emotion underlying CBT (Beck, 1967; Ellis, 1958) describe how an activating event leads to beliefs which in turn leads to emotional and behavioural consequences. The HCBT model contains this idea but also includes the concept of spirit and is less linear and more fluid. It recognises that information is continually being received and responded to at different levels and then further responses are generated from these responses.

External influences

Around the outside of the concentric circles there are five boxes that represent five key areas of external influence. In standard CBT (see Figure 1.1: CBT Formulation on page 19) the past is seen as the main influence that forms core beliefs and the importance of the past is also recognised in this model. However, this model also suggests that other influences (from any of the four other boxes) may also have an impact on the individual and so can modify these core beliefs. For example, a person may have experienced a trauma in their past such as physical or sexual abuse which may lead to them forming beliefs such as the world isn't safe and that people can't be trusted. However, this person may become part of a network with positive social and cultural beliefs which enables them to develop strong, healthy relationships that increases their sense of safety and which helps to modify their initial trauma-based beliefs. These modified beliefs may have as much influence on them as the previous core beliefs from their past trauma and be persistent and pervasive in different areas of the person's life. So, core beliefs in the HCBT model are predominantly developed from the past but can be mediated by the other areas of influence. They are usually beliefs about ourselves, the world, other people and about our future. These beliefs may be out of the person's awareness but they usually strongly influence our psychological responses and behaviours.

Looking at the different external influences, we first have the past, in line with standard CBT. This box relates to core beliefs that develop through early life as a result of how the person interprets childhood events. It may also include genetic factors, such as a family history of psychosis.

The next influence that can contribute to the formation of core beliefs are social influences. This includes systemic ideas that a person is part of their wider social network of family, friends and acquaintances. It focuses on how a person can be influenced by relational issues and processes, particularly from peers and families. This is a reminder that we are social beings and have a built in need to be in social networks, and so an absence of healthy relationships can also lead to unhelpful core beliefs.

There are then cultural influences, and these consist of shared beliefs and behaviours within a culture which can influence a person. As we have already said, culture could include the person's ethnic culture or it could be a culture related to their age group, employment or leisure activities, for example 'NHS culture', 'office culture' or an online gaming culture.

Another influence is the environment. This highlights the influence of our physical surroundings such as our living and working environment. It may include issues beyond the person's control such as local community deprivation and unemployment levels, as well as poorly maintained housing or unethical business environments. Within the area of the environment, HCBT emphasises the value of connecting with nature and how this can support our well-being.

The final box represents spiritual influences and, as discussed in the last chapter, this could include spiritual entities such as a divine being, evil forces, jinn or angels. In the HCBT formulation, the spiritual influences box is available for when people believe that there is a spiritual world that can impact our lives. Acknowledging this within a formulation helps people to voice any spiritual beliefs they may have and acts as a prompt for the therapist to ask about this area. For example, a client may have a sense that God is protecting them and giving them peace, or they may have a fear that jinn are affecting their well-being. So these beliefs can be acknowledged and added to the formulation.

Standard CBT seeks to be collaborative and to create a shared formulation. Yet in standard CBT these ideas would be considered beliefs rather than external influences, which is not then a shared formulation, because for the client it is more than a belief – it is their reality. The therapist does not have to believe that the peace which the person is experiencing is actually from an external deity or that there are jinn affecting their mood, but they can agree to formulate these aspects of a person's life in this way. This then reflects how a person is perceiving the world and makes the formulation truly collaborative.

This model therefore allows people to formulate issues within the worldview which fits the client's spiritual beliefs. If a person is part of a faith community, then this leads to potentially going back to the boxes for the social and cultural influences and exploring these in terms of this faith community. If someone attends a temple, mosque or other place of worship, this is a social event and they are part of a social community. There is also a cultural element to this – such as the temple culture or the church culture, which is also influenced by the ethnicities within the faith community. For example, the culture of a Black Pentecostal church in South London is quite different to the culture of an Anglican parish village church in the home counties, and yet in some assessments they would be both classed as Christian and not explored any further.

As we are assessing these different influences we are being curious about what they are and whether the person feels that they are helping or hindering their well-being and personal growth. This is why it is important to separate out the spiritual, cultural and social elements of a person's faith, for example because someone who is isolated and struggling with mental health difficulties may feel that their prayer life gives a sense of meaning and peace to their life. Socially, they may feel supported by people visiting from their place of worship and knowing that they belong to a group of people that care for them. However, there may also be cultural pressures coming from their faith community that are not so supportive, such as feeling pressure to attend meetings. Therefore, teasing out these three elements of a person's faith can help us to understand their situation better.

We have focused a little more on the spiritual aspect of this model than the other aspects but this is because the other aspects are more familiar, as they are often part of standard CBT. It is the spiritual aspect which is being added to redress a balance. If there are no beliefs in a spiritual world then this is not added to the formulation.

The HCBT model recognises that, as well as being influenced by their culture, environment, social network and the spiritual world, individuals can also have some influence on these different areas (excluding the past, for obvious reasons). In some cases, the influence they exert may be small compared to the influence on them, but the model recognises that the individual is an agent of change. This level of influence is represented by the smaller arrows in the diagram. For example, an individual can make changes to their home environment or in relationships in order to change the impact these have on their well-being. So there is an ongoing, fluid relationship both within the individual, between the different areas of a person, and also between the person and the context in which they live.

It is also important to recognise that the sources of influence can be both helpful and unhelpful in terms of managing a particular presenting problem. The areas of influence could have led to unhelpful core beliefs and may trigger unhelpful responses, but they can also be sources of help. This is one reason why it is useful to identify areas of influence in a person's life so that they can explore what helps and what hinders them with their particular issues that they are bringing to therapy. For example, someone growing up with OCD (Obsessive Compulsive Disorder) may have a family which is both a helpful and unhelpful social influence. The family could be very supportive and understanding, which is a helpful social influence in terms of developing core beliefs of self-worth and knowing they are loved. However, due to the family's concern, they may develop habits that support the maintenance of the OCD. These could include giving reassurance whenever asked for and helping the person with their checking behaviours. These actions are formulated as unhelpful social influences.

This model may not feel too dissimilar to standard CBT and often all these influences are assessed and explored within standard CBT. However, by labelling them in a more explicit model, it ensures that they are directly explored. This ensures that the person is not formulated in isolation, devolved from their wider context.

The multifaceted glass lantern

Symbolism and analogy can be useful tools, particularly when we are trying to describe something so abstract as personhood and trying to define a model of self. In reality we are so complex that no simple model can fully describe our complexity, but the analogy of a lantern offers us a useful way of visualising the HCBT model. Picture a glass lantern made up of different coloured pieces of glass with a candle inside, such as the one in Figure 2.3: Lantern.

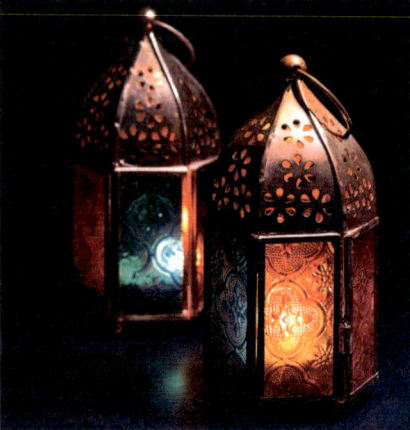

Figure 2.3: Lantern

Firstly, the lantern has a frame, which represents the physical body giving the external shape and form of the individual – creating a container for the other parts. The lantern's frame represents our unique physical identity. This includes such aspects as our eye colour and body form, even down to the shape of our ears and nose. All these aspects are developed from a combination of our genes, our environment, how we care for our body as well as the amazing biology within each of us. The glass panels, meanwhile, represent our psychological aspects and are made up of different shapes and colours that reflect our character, interests, choices and psychological uniqueness. And finally there is the human spirit, which is represented by the lit candle at the heart of the lantern and is the spiritual part of our identity. This candle brings life to the whole structure and helps to enliven and enrich the coloured glass. We will return to this lantern analogy in Chapter 4 when we look at the developmental model of HCBT.

HCBT Longitudinal formulation

In CBT we often use what are called longitudinal formulations, similar to Figure 1.1: CBT Formulation in Chapter 1 (see page 19). CBT formulations show how problems have developed over time and also what is currently maintaining them. Traditionally, CBT formulations have been used to collate the different aspects that have led to a particular problem, and then the formulation is used as guidance for the therapy. Figure 2.4: HCBT formulation shows the generic longitudinal HCBT formulation. (An example of a personalised HCBT formulation is in Chapter 5, on page 114, which describes a case study of individual HCBT.) The formulation in HCBT is not just focused on the problem but also includes strengths and helpful patterns that could act as resources in the therapy. For this reason, the formulation contains both helpful and unhelpful cycles because it is looking at solutions as well as just understanding the problem. Clients who can identify helpful influences and helpful cycles seem to be more likely to visualise themselves acting in positive ways. Having these helpful cycles therefore strengthens the likelihood that a person will move towards more helpful patterns of behaviour and healthier versions of self.

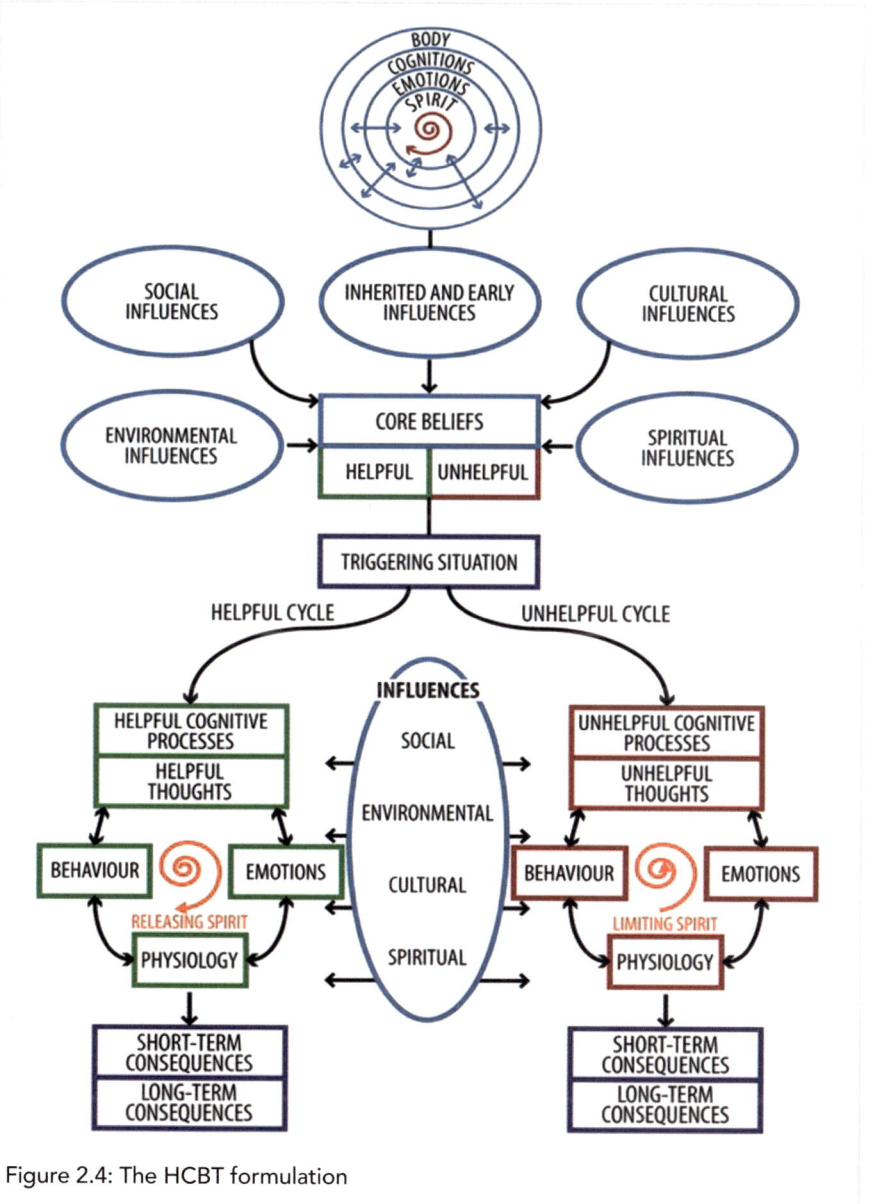

Figure 2.4: The HCBT formulation

The more holistic the longitudinal formulation is, the more complex it becomes, so this formulation can initially look a bit complicated. However, it is offered as a guide, or a road map, to help keep a more holistic view in mind. As with all formulations, it is to be used as a basic guide in order to cover the key topics within therapy and suggests how these aspects may inter-relate. It is not the aim of HCBT to be used in such a manualised way that these formulations become generic and uniform. This formulation template is to be used as a basis to be adapted in order to create personalised formulations that reflect the individual's situation and unique identity.

This formulation is based on the standard CBT formulations. However, the model adds the person in the form of the HCBT model at the beginning of the formulation. It makes the assumption that a person is born with a spirit, along with the more obvious psychological and physical aspects of an individual. The person then develops, and a range of influences affect them leading to core beliefs that can be helpful or unhelpful in terms of a particular presenting problem. As you can see within this formulation, the core beliefs are defined by past experiences, which is the same as with standard CBT. However, the holistic CBT model expands this, as we have already seen, to suggest that there are different areas to be considered within the general umbrella of 'the past'. It is hoped that in good CBT the therapist is able to draw out these different aspects. However, the HCBT model helps to elaborate on the past by explicitly asking about inherited factors and early influences along with cultural, social, spiritual and environmental influences. By identifying these various past influences, the client is more likely to be seen within a wider context rather than in isolation as tends to happen when these factors are grouped under a heading of 'the past' in standard CBT.

These four main areas of influence (excluding inherited and early influences) are also included in the second part of the formulation to acknowledge ongoing influences which may be the same or different to the past influences. So, as already mentioned, this model acknowledges that the past has a profound impact on people, particularly when they are in their formative years. Yet the model also acknowledges current influences that can shape and alter these earlier perceptions of the world, themselves and others. There will be situations in which an influence is in both a person's past and current situation, such as a cultural or family influence. In this case, the participant needs to decide in which box the issue is best placed, according to their understanding of the degree of influence; whether it is more from their past or more of a current cultural influence. Alternatively, it can be put as both past and current influences. However, the important point is to identify the influence rather than become overly concerned as to which box it should be placed in.

Trigger situations for a person's problems are identified, which could include internal, social, cultural, environmental or spiritual triggers. The model then suggests that the trigger can lead to either an unhelpful cycle of unhelpful responses, or a helpful cycle of helpful responses. In reality, there could be a range of responses, but to simplify the model two main possibilities are identified within the therapy, one helpful and one unhelpful.

The cycles are similar to the traditional CBT 'hot cross bun model' (Greenberger & Padesky, 1995) but they separate the 'thoughts' box into two sections: the cognitive processes and the thoughts themselves. This acknowledgement of cognitive processes is based on ideas from metacognitive therapy (Wells & Matthews, 1994) and might include cognitive processes such as worry and rumination in the unhelpful cycles and mindfulness in the helpful cycle. The elements of the helpful and unhelpful cycles interact in the same way that would be proposed by standard CBT. However, in each cycle there is the addition of the spirit which can also influence the different parts of the cycles.

In the unhelpful cycle, where there are unhelpful reactions to the trigger situation, the spirit is more limited and is represented in the diagram as an inwardly spiralling arrow. This unhelpful cycle can distance the individual from their own strengths and potential and so reinforces their unhelpful patterns of thoughts and behaviours, limiting the spirit. These unhelpful cycles, if repeated over time, can develop into more fixed patterns of unhealthier versions of self.

To move from the unhelpful cycle to the helpful cycle, the person needs to be able to start recognising what is happening and to detach themselves from that spiralling process of unhelpful thoughts and behaviours. One of the ways this can be done is by stilling the negative cycling through connecting with the still centre, the spirit. The person can then start to move away from the unhelpful cycle and to begin responding in more helpful ways, within the helpful cycle.

In the helpful cycle the person is thinking and behaving in more helpful ways, their spirit is more free. Over time, if these cycles are repeated, the core essence of the person is liberated, which in turn helps them to have more helpful thoughts and behaviours. The spirit in this cycle is represented by an outwardly spiralling arrow. The individual becomes more free to be themselves, hence the HCBT course name 'Free to be Me'. The formulation therefore highlights the choice of how to respond to the triggering situation. As the founder of logotherapy, psychiatrist Victor Frankl, says:

> 'Between stimulus and response there is a space. In that space is our power to choose our response. In our response lies our growth and our freedom.' (Frankl, 1959)

The spirit can be a resource and can act as an inner compass. Part of HCBT is about helping people to learn to listen more to their spirit and to recognise what most resonates with them. This in turn helps them to recognise what helps to strengthen their healthier self. Their spirit can provide an inner resolve and source of self-compassion to help bring about helpful cycles and helpful responses instead of unhelpful ones. It therefore strengthens the helpful processes in order to develop and strengthen the healthier self. However, HCBT does not dictate how people should connect with their spirit in any particular way and tries not to define it too strictly. So although it uses the term 'spirit', it can be used with anyone because the person can choose how to define spirit according to their own belief system. (We will explore this further in the next chapter.) The formulation is therefore a template on which people can add their own experiences and use their own language, particularly regarding the term 'spirit'. In therapy it is important to use the client's language to fit with their understanding, changing the term 'spirit' to terms such as 'identity', 'consciousness', 'heart' or 'self'.

The core beliefs and cycles are divided into helpful and unhelpful aspects, which encourages a more balanced focus on both. The formulation uses colour coding to make this clearer, with red representing unhelpful and green representing helpful. As with standard CBT, the cycles then lead to short-term and long-term consequences. As Aristotle said:

> 'We are what we repeatedly do; excellence then is not an act, but a habit.'

So, for example, if we are continually living in an unhelpful cycle of social anxiety then we may start avoiding places that make us anxious. This can initially help us to feel safer. This avoidance and sense of safety are the short-term consequences of the unhelpful anxiety cycle. However, in the long-term this cycle reinforces our sense of isolation and the fear of what others might think of us. Over time we become an anxious person and this is the defined role that we identify with and how others perceive us. This becomes an unhealthy version of ourselves. Alternatively, if, to quote a book title, we 'feel the fear and do it anyway' (Jeffers, 2007), we choose to go out and meet people then we develop a helpful cycle. This would lead to short-term consequences of feeling good at mastering something that we had been avoiding. Gradually over time we would grow in confidence and have a role that is outgoing and sociable. So, if we develop more helpful cycles then in the long-term we are developing a healthier version of our self.

Ideally, the aim is to recognise when we are moving into an unhelpful cycle and instead of circling round this unhelpful cycle, we seek to connect with our centre, our spirit, in order to refocus and respond from this still place. When we do this, we then start to move into a helpful cycle and this will then lead to a positive circling. We will start to manage the situation in more healthy ways, experiencing helpful thoughts leading to helpful behaviours and emotions.

When the terms helpful and unhelpful are used in HCBT, this is in terms of what moves a person to greater wholeness and well-being and being who they are within their spirit. So having doubts and questions about an issue may feel negative and unsettling but may not be labelled as unhelpful. If they lead to a greater self-awareness and well-being then they would be seen as helpful thoughts.

The aim of the HCBT formulation is to bring together different aspects of a person's life and to formulate how that person has developed. The formulation is therefore used as a basis from which to ask questions and to consider different areas to form an individualised formulation. Some people may not identify things to go into every box in the formulation. And some things could be written repeatedly in a number of the boxes. This doesn't matter and it is less important to have the right things in the right boxes than to have everything included in at least one of the boxes. This builds an accurate overall picture of the person in relation to a particular triggering situation for a presenting difficulty. The formulation is a tool or springboard for the individual to reflect on different aspects of their life rather than a protocol that has to be adhered to strictly.

Helpful and unhelpful cycle formulations

Often in CBT we don't use the full longitudinal formulation with clients and we may instead draw current maintenance cycles. So let's take the example of a basic CBT cycle for someone who is socially anxious. If we incorporate the spirit alongside unhelpful thoughts, emotions and action, then the cycle for anxiety becomes like the one shown in Figure 2.5: Unhelpful cycle for anxiety.

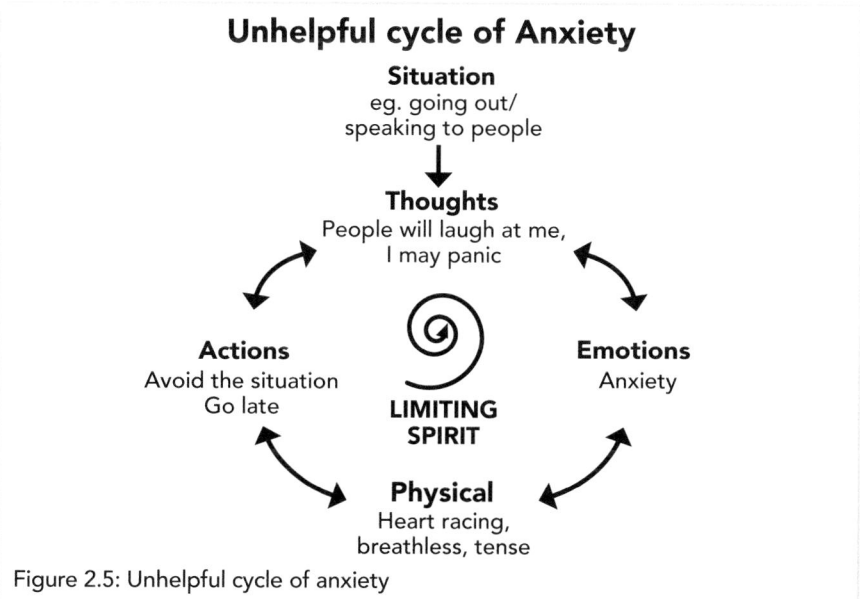

Figure 2.5: Unhelpful cycle of anxiety

If we were to draw a helpful cycle of this situation, it would have the spirit at the centre becoming more free. In return, the spirit then helps to strengthen that cycle, and so the helpful cycle looks like the one in Figure 2.6: Helpful cycle of anxiety.

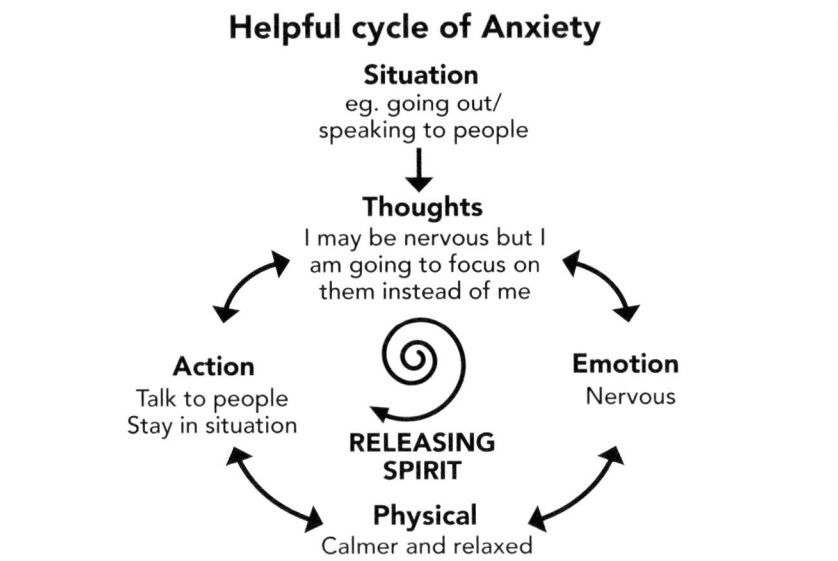

Figure 2.6: Helpful cycle of anxiety

As with any CBT model, these formulations are simplified representations and relate to just one type of trigger whereas in reality there are numerous cycles that are triggered by numerous events and situations. These diagrams can help us to acknowledge the different aspects of ourselves but in reality these parts are all intertwined and inseparable. In practice, we are moving between multiple layers of thoughts and behaviour every moment and these are made up of a complex mixture of helpful and unhelpful cycles. Some of these cycles are within our awareness and some are beyond our awareness. However, they all still impact us and would be more accurately shown as a mesh of interacting cycles of helpful and unhelpful responses. The boxes and cycles of the formulations can help us to keep the different aspects in mind and can act as a checklist to ensure that we don't overlook certain aspect of a person's life.

Those cyclical patterns which are out of our awareness could be seen as similar to the psychodynamic idea of the shadow. We can learn to gradually recognise these unhelpful patterns so that we can begin to change them. As well as more unhelpful patterns, there may also be helpful patterns that are also out of our awareness. Those helpful cycles outside of our awareness could be seen to relate to the psychoanalytical idea of 'the gold in the shadow'. By recognising these helpful cycles we can be more intentional in using them in order to move to a healthier version of our self.

The Free to be Me course

The HCBT model is the basis for the Free to be Me course. This is a personal development course with a psychoeducational approach. It consists of 16 sessions which are described in detail in the companion *Free to be Me* manual. The programme can be used as an individual approach though it is recommended as a group process. Over the weeks the group participants go through each different part of the formulation to develop their own personalised longitudinal formulation. The sessions are:

Session 1: What's this all about?
Session 2: How do I feel?
Session 3: What do I think?
Session 4: Who am I?
Session 5: Where am I going?
Session 6: What do I do?
Session 7: How can I start to change?
Session 8: How can I think differently to feel better?
Session 9: How can I act differently to feel better?
Session 10: How much do I care for my body?
Session 11: How has my past affected me?
Session 12: What about others in my life?
Session 13: How does my environment affect my well-being?
Session 14: How do my beliefs affect my well-being?
Session 15: How can I find balance?
Session 16: How does this all fit together?

Tree as a symbol of spirit

The HCBT formulation is made in two parts: the longitudinal HCBT model, which we have just explored, and the tree picture. The tree is used as a symbol of our spirit and is a way of focusing in on the spirit within the wider HCBT model. Within the longitudinal formulation the spiral represents the spirit and is therefore representative of the tree, shown in Figure 2.5: The spirit within the HCBT Formulation. The tree is drawn and developed throughout the Free to be Me course. It provides a way to help people to reflect on their understanding of their spirit as part of the longitudinal formulation.

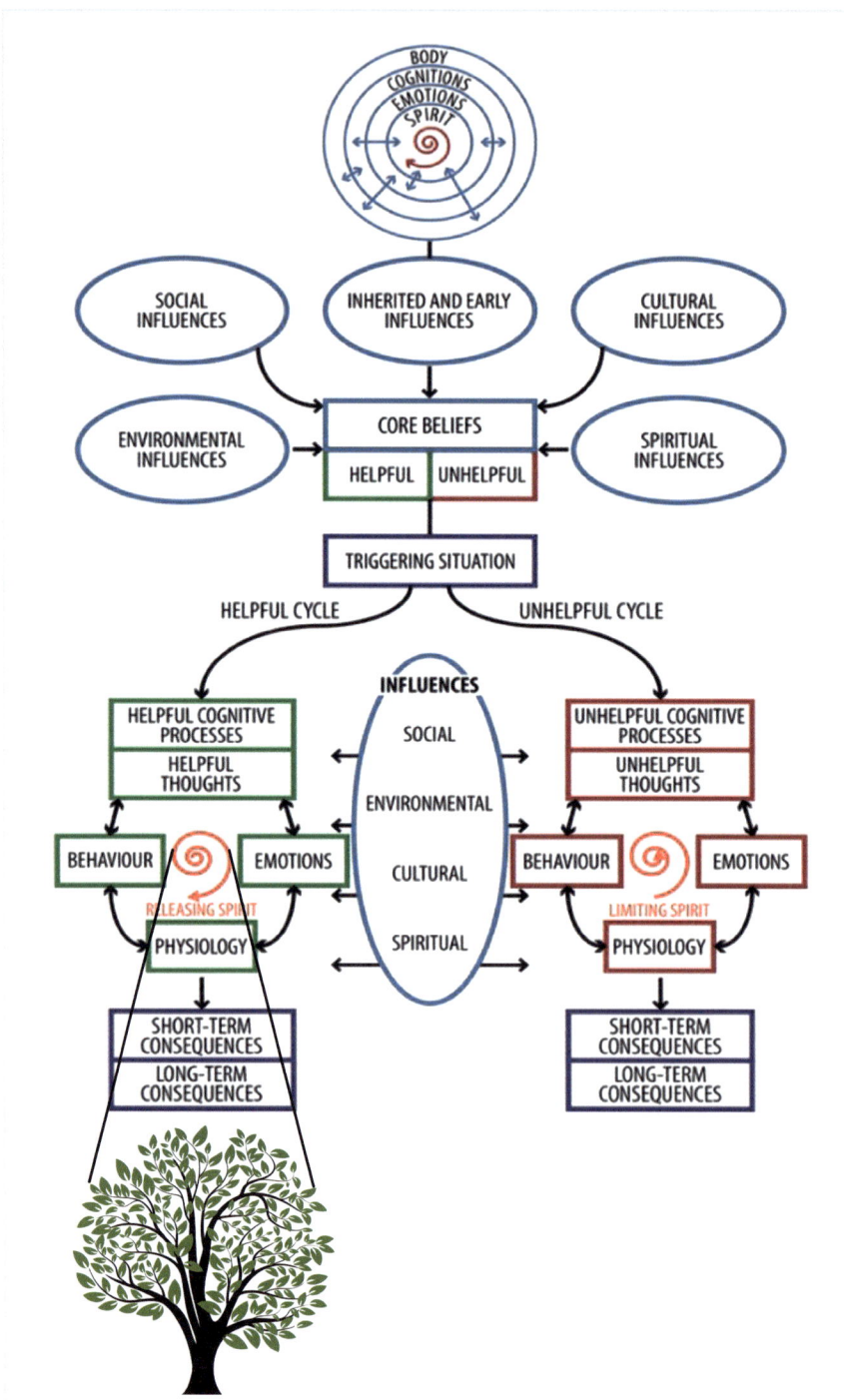

Figure 2.5: The spirit within the HCBT Formulation

The concept of spirit or identity is quite hard to pin down and so the image of a tree is used to help with this process. On the Free to be Me course, people are asked to choose an image of a tree from various photographs. They then discuss what resonates with them about their tree picture. Later in the same session they each draw a tree while reflecting on who they are, and this image may be related to the photo they originally chose. During the course sessions, different aspects of the tree are drawn and labelled. This leads to a final tree picture which is a visual representation of their spirit and what might strengthen or come from their spirit. The tree acts as a way of identifying different aspects of themselves which form or resonate with their spirit (see Figure 2.6: Aspects of The Tree Diagram). There is also a communal tree which is drawn collectively as a group.

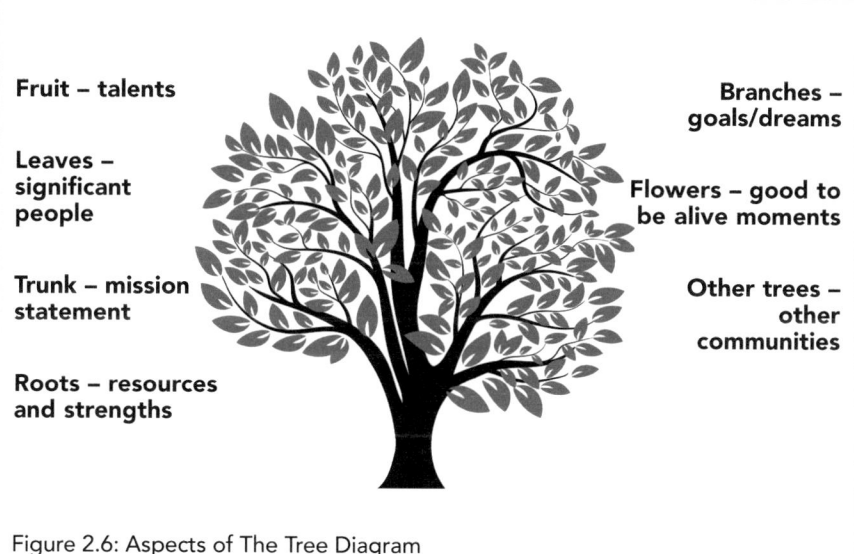

Figure 2.6: Aspects of The Tree Diagram

The tree is made up of the roots, which represent our resources and what keeps us grounded; the branches are our dreams and goals; the fruit are our achievements and talents; the leaves represent significant and supportive relationships; the flowers or blossom represent fun or meaningful moments which make us glad to be alive and the trunk which is our mission or life purpose. We also identify the communities to which we belong, by drawing other trees in the picture. This tree image has similarities to the images used in the Tree of Life groups (Ncube, 2006). However, Ncube used the tree symbol as a narrative approach specifically for trauma work and to reflect people's recovery journey. The HCBT tree image of the spirit was developed independently at a similar time to Ncube's work, and though there are overlapping features, it represents something different.

Trees are a good symbol for the spirit for so many reasons. They are totally international and in many ancient and religious traditions they are seen as symbolic of strength, life and stability. They symbolise uniqueness, for although trees can be of a certain species they are each unique with different shapes and branches. They offer a lot of valuable symbolism as part of the Free to be Me course, such as their beauty even when they are broken or moss covered. The markings on them reflect the tree's life events leaving scars and knots on the bark that are unique to each specimen. There is also the wonderful imagery of trees just being who they are meant to be – not striving to produce fruit but just doing so as part of their lives. In her book *Think Like a Tree: The natural principles guide to life*, Sarah Spencer gives some powerful insights and lessons from the life of trees such as their resilience and the importance of interconnectedness (Spencer, 2019). Figure 2.7: Tree example shows an example of a tree drawn on the course (adapted to maintain anonymity) and there is another example in Chapter 5.

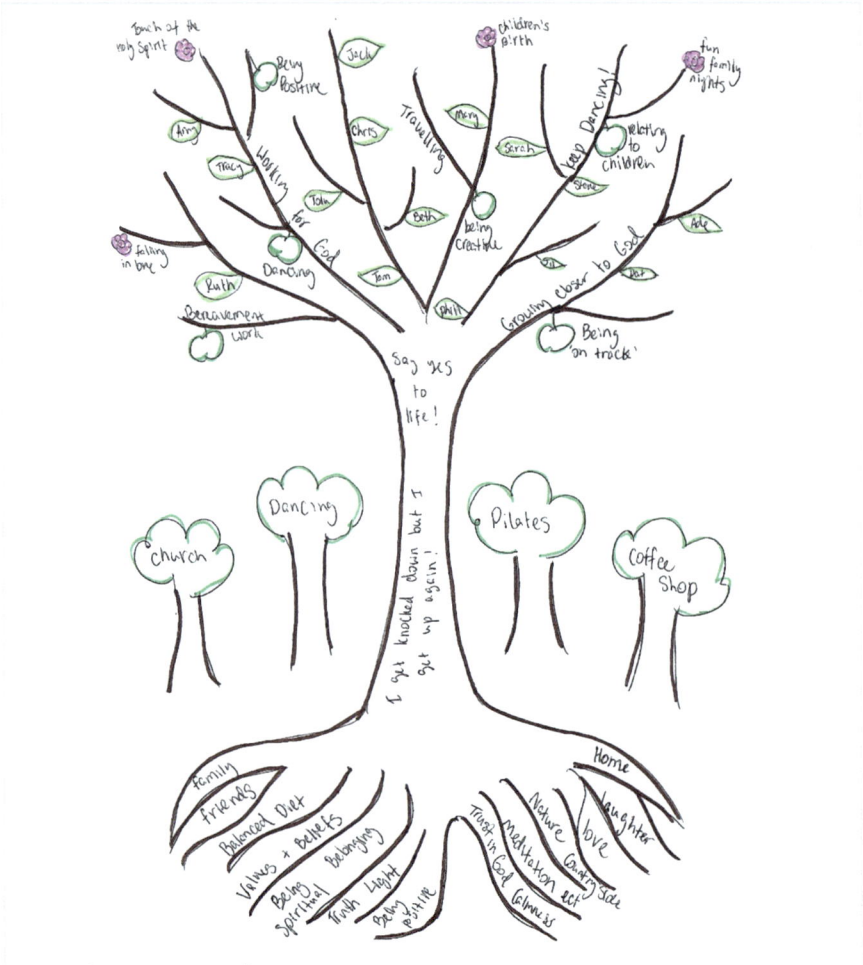

Figure 2.7: Tree example

Outcomes

To date we can only offer small scale outcome data based on the Free to be Me courses run so far. Ideally, we hope to run some research trials in the future on HCBT, in order to collect more large-scale data. Over the different Free to be Me groups we have tried using different outcome measures so we do not have comparable data for all groups run. However, we have now settled on using three outcome measures, along with qualitative data: the Patient Health Questionnaire (PHQ-9 for depression, Spitzer, 1999), the Generalised Anxiety Disorder Assessment (GAD-7 for anxiety, Spitzer *et al*, 2006), and the Shortened Warwick-Edinburgh Mental Well-being Scale (SWEMWBS for general well-being, Tennant *et al*, 2007). We consistently see improvements in all three measures and Table 2.1 shows outcomes for 12 participants who made up the last two groups. One group was in an NHS secondary care mental health setting and one in a community setting. Similar scores were also seen for an online version of the group which was run during the Covid-19 'lockdown' period.

Table 2.1: Scores for outcome measures

Outcome measure	Pre mean score	Post mean score	Mean improvement
PHQ-9	13.8	9.1	4.7
GAD-7	14	10	4
SWEMWBS	28.6	33.8	5.2

A consistent outcome is the level of attendance which appears to be higher than average compared to other CBT groups within NHS settings. This is especially encouraging considering that this course of 16 sessions is longer than standard CBT groups, which often have about 6-12 sessions. The first Free to be Me course was run with a group recruited from a community mental health team in an East London NHS service and consisted of eight participants. The dropout rate was zero with an average attendance of 74%.

At the end of each course participants have attended a focus group and the recorded data has been analysed using Interpretative Phenomenological Analysis. Once we have gathered more data, we plan to publish the results of identified themes along with the improvements shown in the outcome measures. Unsurprisingly, some themes already emerging are typical for standard CBT groups such as the value of being in a group, the value of recognising maintenance cycles and making cognitive and behavioural changes. However, there are other themes more typical to this course such as valuing the use of creativity; seeing the therapeutic value of connecting with nature; valuing the recognition of spirituality in relation to mental health and becoming more aware of a person's individuality and strengths.

Chapter 3: Our human spirit

The concept of the Human spirit

In developing HCBT, the concepts of identity and spirituality could not easily be aligned to the existing standard parts of a CBT formulation, namely thoughts, emotions, behaviours and physical sensations. The model needed something that reflected the person as a whole and something that seemed to go deeper than these different parts of a person's psychology. In listening to clients talk about their experiences, they often describe strong emotions and strongly held beliefs. Yet there is also something deeper than this that sometimes seems to be the source of these strong convictions or passions. This source can seem to be at the heart of who they are; it is about a deeper knowing, a sense of conscience or intrinsic sense of self. These ideas seem to fit with the concept of the human spirit. The other aspects of the HCBT formulation are more familiar to us and easier to define. So this chapter will offer some thoughts about how to define and connect with this obscure concept of our human spirit.

The English language uses many phrases that refer to our spirit, such as 'this person is very high spirited'; 'they had a strong spirit that got them through'; 'they've got a lot of spirit'; and 'she is a free spirit'. According to the Collins dictionary the term 'spirit' can refer to the following:

> 'The human spirit is virtually indestructible; A person's spirit is the non-physical part of them that is believed to remain alive after their death; A spirit is a ghost or supernatural being; Spirit is the courage and determination that helps people to survive in difficult times and to keep their way of life and their beliefs; Spirit is the liveliness and energy that someone shows in what they do. The spirit in which you do something is the attitude you have when you are doing it; A particular kind of spirit is the feeling of loyalty to a group or a set of ideas, beliefs and aims that is shared by the people who belong to the group; the spirit of something such as a law or an agreement is the way that it was intended to be interpreted or applied; You can refer to a person as a particular kind of spirit if they show a certain characteristic or if they show a lot of enthusiasm in what they are doing. Your spirits are your feelings at a particular time, especially feelings of happiness or unhappiness.' (Collins, online)

Related to the term 'spirit', is the term 'self', and the philosopher and early psychologist William James described the mental self as:

> '…the active element of all consciousness … the central active self … the very core and nucleus of our self, as we know it, the very sanctuary of our life, is the sense of activity which certain inner states possess. The sense of activity is often held to be a direct revelation of the living substance of our soul.' (James, 1890)

This idea is also explored by the philosopher Galen Strawson, who described the mental self as:

> '…a mental presence; a mental someone; a single mental thing that is a conscious subject, that has a certain character or personality, and that is distinct from all its particular experiences, thoughts, hopes, wishes, feelings and so on.' (Strawson, 2017)

There are also arguments to say that there is no such thing as a spirit, or a self, as expressed in the writings of the philosophers Daniel Dennett and Anthony Kenny. In his book *The Self*, Kenny argues that the self is a self-constructed concept and a 'grammatical illusion', saying that:

> 'The psychological root of the notion of the self derives from the idea that imagination is an interior sense… The self is the eye of inner vision, the ear of inner hearing or rather it is the mythical possessor of both inner eye and inner ear and whatever other inner organs of sensation may be fantisized.' (Kenny, 1988)

Even though there may be some debate as to whether such an entity actually exists, the spirit is nevertheless a useful concept therapeutically, and one to which many relate.

Ancient understandings of spirit

Historically, the Ancient Greeks had a range of beliefs about the spirit, or what they sometimes called the soul. The philosopher Socrates famously said, 'to know thyself is the beginning of wisdom', and he taught that 'thyself' was made up of both body and soul. He taught that the soul was an immortal, immaterial entity within each of us and that the body and soul form an undivided unity that could only be separated at death. These teachings set the foundation for Western dualistic thinking of body and soul, which were further developed by 17th-century French philosopher Descartes, who proposed that everything can be divided into either matter or spirit.

Returning to Ancient Greece, Socrates described the concept of a 'daimon', or 'god within', which he saw as an internal guide or divine conscience. Greek philosophers encouraged their students to live according to their 'daimon' – or true self – in order to reach their potential and fulfil what they were each capable of. One image that was used to illustrate this was how a potter made a clay pot on a potter's wheel. The clay begins at the centre of the wheel and is formed from the centre illustrating the idea that our true self is at our centre and we are formed from this central place.

Plato developed Socrates' teaching saying that the soul was divided into three parts: reason, desires and spirit. He described the spirit as being willpower and energy and that a healthy soul is when the spirit controls the desires with reason, and the three work in harmony with each other. So, Plato compared this process to being like a charioteer who was trying to control two horses. Plato's student, Aristotle, challenged his ideas about the soul and said that reason is not about suppressing desires but about directing and guiding them. Aristotle talked about the soul being the life within something and the capacity it has to fulfil their potential. He described how everything has a soul; it was possible to have a vegetable soul and an animal soul as well as the human soul. For Aristotle, then, an oak tree's soul is its ability and life to make it grow and bear acorns and, in the same way, a human soul gives us the capacity to be who we truly are.

Aristotle developed Socarates idea of the 'daimon' and taught that 'eudaimonia' was achieved when we acted according to one's 'daimon' – living from the divine wisdom at our centre. This idea of eudaimonia closely relates to the positive psychology concepts of flourishing, intrinsic motivation and flow, and Maslow's concept of self-actualisation (which we will return to when we explore humanism later in this chapter). The Greek philosophers differentiated eudaimonia from hedonism, where the former relates to feelings of being truly alive and being who you really are, as compared to passing pleasures and enjoyment. Plutarch, another Greek philosopher, pictured the soul as a weaver who weaves our past into a coherent story so that we have a sense of self and an understanding of who we are.

Stoicism was a significant philosophy at this time and became a key foundation for modern-day CBT. The freed Roman slave Epictetus, who became a stoic philosopher, believed that the concept of the self helped to develop a sense of freedom. Having been a slave himself, he taught that a person's spirit could be free even if his body was enslaved. Within stoicism there was the idea that the universe was created and interconnected through a divine intelligence or 'logos'. The Stoics taught that each person had a spark of this divine intelligence. The Stoic philosophers encouraged people to use this divine intelligence or reason to follow their true nature and that this was the key to fulfilment. The Stoics described how a person has a unique set of qualities which remain consistent throughout their life. This set of qualities makes up the person's forming principle, making them that particular individual. This means that they could be recognised regardless of age, throughout their life.

The concept of the heart was used by many Greek teachers to represent a place of integration within body and soul, and to describe the spiritual centre of a person. The heart was therefore seen as the meeting place between the human and the divine. This use of the term 'heart' has similarities to the Eastern concept of 'chakras', which are centres of the spiritual energy or life force, sometimes known as 'Chi'.

Spirit within psychology

Moving to our modern-day study of psychology, the term 'psychology' is based on the Greek word 'psyche', which means 'spirit, soul or self'. So psychology began as the study of the 'spirit', though it has moved on to the scientific study of the mind and brain as well as many other related areas of study. The transpersonal psychologist and philosopher Ken Wilber reflected on how this change of focus may have limited our understanding of human potential and personhood:

> '…the roots of modern psychology lie in spiritual traditions and the study of psychology ought ideally to be the study of all of that, body to mind to soul.' (Wilber, 2000)

Wilber advocates for a return to ancient wisdom and an integrated understanding of spirit and matter as inseparable, and that:

> '…these pioneering modern psychologists (referencing Fechner, James and Baldwin) managed to be both fully scientific and fully spiritual and they found not the slightest contradiction in that generous embrace.' (Wilber, 2000)

Within my own work, I have taught on integrating spirituality within therapy over a number of years in different settings. This has often been with trainee or qualified psychologists but also with other mental health workers from varied professions and backgrounds. Within this teaching I have asked, 'What comes to mind when you hear the term 'spirit' in terms of a person's human spirit?' There is often a lot of overlap and consistency between answers, and these are the responses collected so far:

- Heart or core of a person, the positive potential within us.
- Breath of life, life force, essence.
- 'Soul', connects with God or part of God, a divine spark, God within.
- True self, real identity, unique individual, constant part of self.
- State of flow, of doing something that comes naturally, absorbed in the moment, energising.
- Inner resolve/driving force to keep going in a difficult situation, strength to stay alive, to keep fighting.

- Inner wisdom/gut instinct/conscience/values/Wise Mind (from DBT).
- The source of deepest dreams, ambitions, motivations, values, destiny, purpose and meaning.
- The place in which I feel a connection/oneness/sense of belonging with others/natural world/ancestors/universe/God.
- The observing self (from mindfulness or ACT).
- Energy/auras.
- Non-physical part of a person/immortal/ghost/eternal.
- Higher or deeper levels of consciousness/awareness/where we 'know that we know'/ consciousness of being/intuition.
- Mystery/cannot quantify/intangible.

Although there is sometimes a different language or terminology used, there seems to be a core understanding of what we mean by our human spirit. This concept seems to resonate with people and therefore seemed a useful concept to add to the CBT formulation to represent a person's identity and what is deepest within us.

The human spirit has been defined as:

> '…the dynamic force that keeps a person growing and changing, continuously involved in a process of emerging, becoming and transcending of self.' (Goddard, 1995)

Another definition describes the spirit as that which:

> '…enables and motivates us to search for meaning and purpose in life, to seek the supernatural or some meaning which transcends us, to wonder about our origins and our identities, to require morality and equality. It is the spirit which synthesizes the total personality and provides some sense of energizing direction and order.' (Ellison, 1983)

HCBT therefore sees an individual as having three integrated parts: the physical, the psychological and the spiritual. People use different terminology such as 'soul', 'higher consciousness', 'true self' or 'heart' when referring to what HCBT terms the 'spirit'. In talking with different people about this concept, there are repeated themes which emerge: the spirit being a source of energy and the potential of who we are; the source of deepest passions and dreams; the foundation of the true self as opposed to false selves. It also conveys something about connection; the part of us that connects most deeply with the spirit of the other and connects to what is beyond ourselves such as the natural world, or perhaps with a spiritual world. People describe stories of resilience in the face of trauma and describe how their spirit, this spark of life, helped to give them hope to survive. People tend to talk about it as a constant aspect of themselves which is intrinsically good. It therefore seems different to the concept of a personality or character, which can have both positive and negative characteristics. People talk about being broken in spirit or that it can be dampened or hidden. The spirit can also be seen as the source of growing consciousness. It is also seen as a source of compassion and gives encouragement to see the potential both within themselves and in others. It is also described as the place where things resonate deeply; that we just know in our spirit that a direction seems right and when it feels more than just a cognitive decision but more a 'gut feeling'.

These ideas are found in the shared ancient wisdom of many faith traditions, sometimes known as the perennial tradition. These traditions teach that within our physical bodies there is something more than the psychological aspect of a person's thoughts and feelings; that there is a spiritual aspect to ourselves too. Within these faith traditions is the idea that there is something of the sacred within us and that through this we are all connected with each other, and with the Sacred. The perennial tradition teaches that life is ultimately about discovering this sacred connection. The concept of the human spirit is shared not only across the main faith traditions but is also recognised, perhaps in a different form, by those who do not adhere to a particular faith tradition, such as the humanistic sense of a shared humanity or a source of inner strength. Roger Walsh explores spiritual practices from the different faith traditions in his book *Essential Spirituality*. He summarises the message of these wisdom traditions saying:

> '…their central message is the same: You are more than you think! Look deep within, and you will find that your ego is only a tiny wave atop the vast ocean that is your real Self … that this Self is intimately linked to the sacred, and that you share in the unbounded bliss of the sacred.' (Walsh, 2000)

The transpersonal psychologist John Rowan describes the 'still small voice of conscience' (Rowan, 2005). This inner voice leads to a vocation, a sense of calling, and helps in making important life decisions (Rowan, 1993). Fabry, another transpersonal psychologist, describes the spirit in this way:

> 'The spirit, like the body and psyche, is part of every person, not just the religiously inclined… It contains our self-detachment or ability to step outside and look at ourselves and our self-transcendence or ability to reach out to people we love and causes in which we believe. In the area of the spirit we are not driven, we are the drivers, the decision makers.' Fabry, 1980)

Although it can be useful to think about separate parts such as the body, mind and spirit, in reality the individual is fully integrated – physical, psychological and spiritual. So the concept of the spirit as a separate entity within the body is artificial in that it cannot be separated from the rest of a person's make up. However, it is a useful concept to recognise as one of the parts which makes the whole. This highlights the importance of holistic thinking recognising that all parts are intricately integrated with each other. This could mean that each part of a person is involved at any one time with any given activity. So an activity cannot be seen as purely psychological and another activity as physical and another as spiritual. For example, praying would not be seen as just a spiritual activity in the same way as eating lunch would not be seen as just a physical activity. Both involve a whole person and so both could be seen as being psychological, physical and spiritual activities. It may be more helpful to think about these three aspects of a person as three windows through which a person is viewed. Whether a person is praying or eating lunch there can be physical, psychological and spiritual aspects to each activity.

Connecting with spirit

In her book *Quiet*, Susan Cain talks about introversion within a world which admires and encourages extraversion. Her concluding chapter begins with this quote from the writer Anais Nin:

> 'Our culture made a virture of living only as extroverts. We discouraged the inner journey, the quest for a centre. So we lost our centre and have to find it again.' (Nin, as quoted by Cain, 2013)

This 'quest for a centre' is potentially about connecting with spirit, and this is one of the things that draws people towards spirituality. So the concept of spirituality naturally develops from that of spirit, and spirituality has been defined as:

> '…the specific way in which individuals and communities respond to the experience of the spirit. Spirituality is how we express our spirit. Spirituality involves a quest for meaning and strives to answer deep existential questions pertaining to the meaning of life, suffering and so forth.' (Swinton, 2001)

In the same way that people describe the spirit in different ways, people find individual ways to express their spirituality. As we have already explored in Chapter 1, for some people spirituality is about being part of a faith tradition, but for others it may be about connecting with others or a sense that life is sacred. Spiritual practices may therefore involve a diverse range of activities such as connecting with nature, praying, serving the local community, creating music and art, yoga and meditation. Others may connect most spiritually with sport; standing singing a football anthem with thousands of fellow supporters is very much a spiritual experience of deep connection, hope and purpose for many. Those of us who have been stirred by a powerful film, play or great novel would have had what Rudolf Otto called 'numinous moments' (Otto, 1923). These are moments when we are connecting with our spirit, when it feels good to be alive, that there is a sense that all is well or that we are experiencing something of wonder and awe. Sometimes it is when we have an experience of deep love or times of severe suffering that we can discover a powerful connection with our spirit. There can be a humbling respect to the mystery and sacredness of life which can come both in profound moments, such as the birth of a child, or more everyday moments such as seeing a breath-taking sunset.

Martsolf and Mickley (1998) identified five central features of spirituality: finding meaning, having values, transcendence beyond the human, connecting with others and connecting with something bigger than ourselves and becoming who you are.

Although there may be some common factors and shared expressions of spirituality, there are individual journeys that are unique to each of us. There is a richness in this diversity and the natural world teaches us that variety is rich and beautiful. There is a danger when we try to reduce that spiritual diversity for people to feel that they can only express their spirituality in certain ways, which limits their self-expression. Instead of celebrating difference; seeing the different spiritual paths and experiences in the same way we might see the beauty of different colours and species in a field of wild flowers. Likewise, the human species is full of diversity and there is a richness in our uniqueness. This is important to celebrate so that we learn from each other rather than insisting that there is one right way to be human.

One way that we can connect with our spirit is being aware of a sense of calling in our lives. A beautifully written book on this topic is *Callings* by Gregg Levoy. He draws from a range of cultural and faith traditions to describe the importance of hearing and following our callings in life. He suggests that if we don't do this then:

> '…we'll feel alienated from ourselves, listless and frustrated and fitful with boredom, the common cold of the soul. Life will feel so penetratingly dull and pointless…' (Levoy, 1997)

He goes on to suggest how we might recognise callings:

> '…whether a particular call has integrity or not, whether it makes us feel more or less authentic, more or less connected to ourselves or others, more or less right, not morally but intuitively… whether a call will give us a feeling of aliveness.' (Levoy, 1997)

He also suggests that we can find our calling by recognising our passions:

> '…what we study when there are no tests to take … it is what we'd do if we weren't worried about consequences, about money, about making anybody happy but ourselves… Passion is the smelling salts of the soul.' (Levoy, 1997)

We can seek to listen to our inner self, our spirit, through various means such as journaling, meditation, therapy, retreats and many other avenues that heighten our self-awareness. Often these practices are about stilling ourselves, and many traditions suggest that it is in silence and meditation that we can best connect with our spirit.

Spirit within different traditions

Let's now briefly look at a few particular ways that the spirit has been understood within different faith traditions and psychological schools of thought. These are just brief introductions; there is not space here to give full justice to each of these rich traditions.

Judaism and Christian tradition

Generally within the Judaism and Christian traditions there is the belief that the soul animates the body and together the body and soul create a united whole.

In Hebrew (the language of the Old Testament and the Jewish tradition), the word used for soul is 'nephesh' meaning 'life' or 'living being'. This is the same word used to describe life within animals, the life force that makes us alive. In the Jewish tradition this life force is in the blood and 'nephesh' is where the spiritual and the physical come together. In the Greek (the language of the New Testament), the word used for soul is 'psyche' from where the word psychology derives its meaning.

The Torah (Jewish scriptures) and the Bible (Christian scriptures) also use a term translated as 'spirit', suggesting this is something more than just our soul or 'psyche'. In Hebrew, the word used is 'ruach' and in Greek it is 'pneuma', but both words can be translated as 'breath' or 'spirit'. This term 'ruach' or 'pneuma' implies energy and being enlivened rather than just being physically alive and conscious, which is implied in the term 'nephesh'.

Within the Jewish tradition there are three levels of our inner self. We have already mentioned the nephesh and ruach, and then the highest level is neshamah. This is a term used to describe the intake of air before it is breathed out – the action needed to create the breath, or ruach. So together these levels of the soul describe the taking in of breath, the breathing out and the bringing to life. This reflects the creation story in the three Abrahamic traditions (Jewish, Christian and Muslim) of God breathing life into Adam, the first man.

So both the Jewish and Christian traditions recognise the spirit as being separate from the psychological and physical aspect of a person. The early church theologian Origen highlighted these three aspects of personhood described in the New Testament: body, soul and spirit, as in the following Bible verse:

> 'Now may the God of peace himself sanctify you completely, and may your whole spirit and soul and body be kept blameless at the coming of our Lord Jesus Christ.' (1 Thessalonians 5 v.23)

And also:

> 'For the word of God is alive and active. Sharper than any double-edged sword, it penetrates even to dividing soul and spirit, joints and marrow.' (Hebrews 4 v.12)

The former chief rabbi in the UK, Rabbi Jonathan Sacks, said:

> 'The resilience of the human spirit … is about the breath of God within us, that helps broken hearts to heal, broken lives to be rebuilt.' (Sacks, 2009)

And in discussing the story of Moses parting the sea, Rabbi Sacks comments:

> 'Just as ruach, a physical wind, can part waters and expose land beneath, so ruach, the human spirit, can expose, beneath the surface of a story, a deeper meaning beneath.' (Sacks, 2017)

In Judaism and Christian traditions, therefore, the human spirit is seen as the breath of God through which God gives life. The name for God in the Jewish tradition is Yahweh, or more accurately the four consonants, YHWH. When this name is spoken it resembles the breathing process and can therefore act as a constant reminder of God breathing life through humanity in the form of the human spirit. Chief Rabbi Dr Warren Goldstein wrote a book entitled *Defending the Human Spirit* in which he describes how the Jewish law:

> '…defends the human spirit – its freedom, creativity and its loftiness and places in order a system that promotes a harmonious society.' (Goldstein, 2005)

In Judaism and Christian traditions the spirit is seen as the invisible, eternal part which can connect a person to God and which makes people spiritual beings. *Genesis* speaks of humanity being made in the image of God. So according to these traditions, people have the potential to discover this image within themselves and in others. Christian traditions in the Western world were influenced by the dualistic Greek thinking of dividing matter and spirit, while the Eastern church retained more of its Jewish roots and the integrated holistic concept of an indivisible body and spirit. A verse suggesting that something of God is within us is from the Jewish Torah (or the Christian Old Testament):

> 'He (God) has made everything beautiful in its time. He has also set eternity in the human heart.' (Ecclesiastes 3 v.11)

Jesus made numerous references to the human spirit, for example, when he was praying through the night in the garden of Gethsemane, his disciples were sleepy and he said to them 'the spirit is willing but the body is weak' (Matthew 26.41). Also when he was dying on the cross Jesus quoted the words of Psalm 31.5 (from the Jewish tradition) saying, 'Into your hands I commit my spirit'.

Paul, one of the first leaders of the early church, wrote that, 'the Spirit testifies with our spirit that we are God's children' (Romans 8 v.16). In this statement, Paul was making the distinction between God, in the form of the Holy Spirit, and the human spirit. The Christian tradition teaches that God lives with the spirit through the Holy Spirit. This enables a person to communicate with God and that gradually the Holy Spirit can change the person to become who God originally created them to be.

Quakers describe the spirit as the 'divine spark' and it has also been described as a seed of God holding the potential to grow into the divine. For example, Meister Eckhart (a 13th century German mystic) said:

> 'The seed of God is in us: Pear seeds grow into pear trees; Hazel seeds into hazel trees; And God seeds into God.'

The Jewish psychiatrist Victor Frankl wrote about his experiences and observations of being in a concentration camp in his book *Man's Search for Meaning*. He shares his experiences and reflections of this time with numerous examples of seeing either his fellow prisoners or himself be sustained by inner strength from their spirit, which for him related to a person's will power. For example, he writes:

> 'Another time we were at work in a trench. The dawn was grey around us; grey was the sky above us; grey the snow in the pale light of dawn; grey the rags in which my fellow prisoners were clad and grey their

faces. In a last violent protest against the hopelessness of imminent death, I sensed my spirit piercing through the enveloping gloom. I felt it transcend that hopeless, meaningless world and somewhere I heard a victorious "Yes" in answer to my question of the existence of an ultimate purpose.' (Frankl, 1959)

Frankl found that those who were able to connect with this inner strength and find meaning in their suffering were able to survive the ordeal. This concept of spirit as inner strength and willpower is seen throughout the Jewish tradition.

Within the mystic and contemplative Christian traditions there are many examples of writings about connecting with our spirit and the belief that this leads to oneness with God through this connection. The monk and contemplative writer Thomas Merton wrote about the concepts of the True self and the False self. He described the True self as 'the deep, transcendent self that awakens in contemplation', and the False self which is, 'the superficial, external self that is not eternal or spiritual.' (Merton, 1962)

Merton described the False self as consisting of default thinking patterns and responses that have developed over the years. In his writings, along with other contemplatives, Thomas Merton described that at the heart of each person is the spirit, which is like the potential of God developing into the True self that could ultimately grow to be one with God. Merton saw contemplation (a form of meditation) as the way to discover this 'ground of our being' within, and to help the True self grow as we gradually let go of the False self.

One of the ways to connect with the spirit that has been used, particularly within the Catholic tradition, is the use of the Examen. This dates back to the 16th century and is part of the Ignatian spiritual exercises. Ignatius of Loyola (the 16th century monk who developed this practice) also talked about the importance of discerning what dreams are within us and the importance of following dreams from the spirit. The Examen encourages people to reflect on each day with two simple questions – what has energised me today and what has drained me? By doing this practice on a regular basis, it helps people to discern what resonates with them and what energises them. This helps to discern what is coming from their spirit and true self. The book *Landmarks*, by Margaret Silf, based on Ignatian spirituality, describes the spirit as a powerful underground stream which is trying to find a way to flow. Silf suggests that we can learn to discern this flow when we see signs of it breaking through onto the surface of our lives. She also describes the spirit as the eye of a storm as well as using the image of an inner compass. She suggests we need to learn to recognise and trust the spirit, suggesting that when we feel we have lost direction we:

'…must come to stillness. In the silence of our hearts, we must wait patiently for the compass needle to steady. Then it will point to true

North, the still centre, the fine point of the soul and we will be enabled to move forward again.' (Silf, 1998)

A significant English mystic who lived at the turn of the 20th century was Evelyn Underhill, who wrote:

'A spiritual life is simply a life in which all that we do comes from the centre, where we are anchored in God.' (Underhill, 1937)

A current Christian contemplative is Richard Rohr. In the following quote he shares his understanding of spirit (which he calls soul), from his book *Falling Upward*:

'I believe that God gives us our soul… our unique blueprint… Our unique little bit of heaven is installed by the Manufacturer within the product, at the beginning! We are given a span of years to discover it … and to live our own destiny to the full. If we do not, our True Self will never be offered again, in our own unique form… The discovery of our soul is crucial and of pressing importance for each of us and for the world. We do not 'make' or 'create' our souls; we just 'grow' them up. We are the clumsy stewards of our own souls. Much of our work is learning how to stay out of the way of this rather natural growing and awakening. We need to unlearn a lot, it seems, to get back to that foundational life… Whether or not we find our True Self depends in large part on the moments of time we are each allotted and the choices we make at those moments. Life is indeed 'momentous', created by accumulated moments in which the deeper 'I' is slowly revealed if we are ready to see it. This is our life's purpose.' (Rohr, 2011)

Islam

The Islamic understanding of the spirit is similar to that of the Judeo-Christian traditions in that God creates the Ruh (spirit) which is similar to the Hebrew word of 'ruach', meaning breath or spirit. Islamic tradition teaches that God breathes this Ruh into a person before birth and the Ruh is believed to live on after the person's death.

Within Islam there are various aspects of a person's internal make up. A helpful diagram to illustrate these different aspects of personhood within the Islamic tradition (Betteridge, unpublished) is shown in Figure 3.1: Basic Islamic concept of the self. The Islamic faith holds that a person is initially born with a spirit that is good and this goodness comes from the Fitra, which is the divine potential to be good. This Fitra is the natural disposition of each person and is a human's innate knowledge of God and how to live. Each person is born with a predisposition to be a Muslim and to grow in the faith which is based on the Fitra, though people may grow up to follow other spiritual traditions, despite this initial predisposition to be Muslim. So according to life's circumstances, the Fitra can be limited and so the person can then become increasingly good or bad depending on what influences the Fitra and how much it is limited. The Fitra, as a concept of inherent goodness, has some parallels with the concept to that of 'spirit' in HCBT.

In the Islamic view of the person's internal makeup there are three other main concepts – the Naffs, the Aql and the Qalb. The Naffs, or soul, are the drives within a person or the life force and is similar to the Jewish understanding of nephesh. The Naffs can also be seen as similar to the concept of the ego. The Aql is the mind and so is the centre of intelligence and reasoning. Thirdly there is the Qalb, which is the heart and the place of deep understanding and emotions, and again the concept of Qalb in Islam has some overlap with the HCBT concept of spirit.

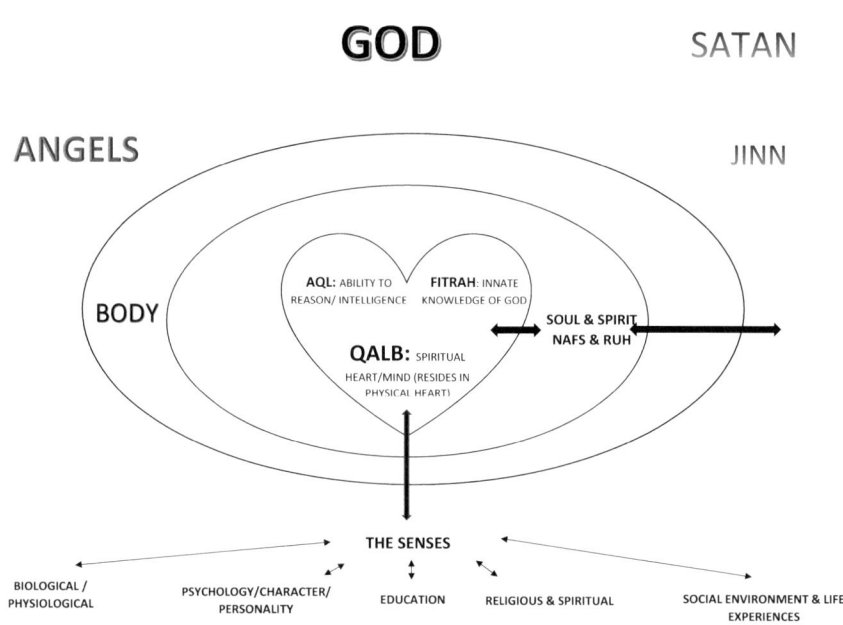

Figure 3.1: Basic Islamic concept of the self

Within the Qalb a person experiences 'God consciousness', which is being aware of and relating to God and is the centre of the Fitra (divine potential). Islamic teachings encourage Muslims to, with God's help, develop the Qalb and so strengthen the Fitra to increase the goodness within the Ruh (spirit).

As the 13th century Sufi mystic Rumi said:

> 'The very centre of your heart is where life begins – the most beautiful place on earth… Everyone has been made for some particular work, and the desire for that work has been put in our heart.' (Rumi)

Hinduism and Sikhism

Hinduism is based on the ancient writings of the Vedas in which a person is described as having three bodies – a gross body, subtle body and causal body. The gross body is the physical body of senses and our physiology. The subtle body consists of the psychological aspects of our intelligence, emotions and our everyday sense of the self. This subtle body gives a person certain auras or energies. The subtle body is seen as being like a force field of energy that is divided into seven levels: physical, etheric, sexual, emotional, astral, mental and psychic. Energy moves round the body through seven different chakras, or energy centres. The causal body is the deepest self and is the ever present consciousness when the gross body and causal body are still. Hinduism teaches that the causal body is the expansive part of ourselves that is uncovered through meditation. The causal body is the source of the person and of the Atman. Atman is the Sanskrit word for spirit and is seen as the true self or essence of a person. So both these concepts of causal body and Atman relate to the HCBT concept of spirit.

The Atman is described as the immortal part of the person that is beyond the mind and senses and is part of God. It gives the person divine qualities such as eternal bliss, honesty, compassion and wisdom, and it also gives the person a reason to exist. It is described as being a flame within the heart and that this self cannot be known intellectually but is only experienced through revelation. A person's soul, or Atman, is believed to have originated in the spiritual world and this is the Atman's ultimate destination. Hinduism encourages detachment from the material world and attachment to God through various spiritual practices. It teaches that a person's real identity is the Atman rather than our body or mind and so spirituality is therefore about discovering and developing this true self.

The traditional Hindu greeting of 'Namaste', which is often used in yoga sessions, acts as a reminder of this internal spirit. Namaste literally means 'the spirit in me greets the spirit in you at the place where we are one'. As one offers this greeting, the hands are held together on the chest which is at the heart centre or 'anahata chakra'.

In a similar way, Sikhs believe that God's spirit lives in each person and this Atma, as it is called in Sikhism, is described as the spiritual spark in the person. The Atma gives life and acts as an internal driver and is described as the 'burning fire of life' (Sri Guru Granth Sahib).

Within Sikhism there is a focus on becoming humble, letting go of the ego and becoming 'Naam'. Naam is a state of true humility in which a person becomes immersed in God and free from pride. Meditation and 'Naam Simran' (loving remembrance of God) is an important part of this process in order to reach a higher consciousness and oneness with God.

In both these religions there is the belief that the spirit moves on to live in another person or animal once the person dies through the process of reincarnation.

In the Hindu scriptures, known as the Upanishads, it says:

> 'You are what your deep, driving desire is. As your desire is, so is your will. As your will is, so is your deed. As your deed is, so is your destiny.' (Brihadaranyaka Upanishad IV.4.5)

The Hindu scriptures describe the spirit (which is translated here using the word soul) in this way:

> 'That which pervades the entire body with consciousness, you should know to be indestructible. No one is able to destroy that imperishable soul … Weapons cannot shred the soul, nor can fire burn it. Water cannot wet it, nor can the wind dry it. The soul is unbreakable and incombustible; it can neither be dampened nor dried. It is everlasting, in all places, unalterable, immutable, and primordial. The soul is spoken of as invisible, inconceivable, and unchangeable. Knowing this, you should not grieve for the body.' (Bhagavad Gita 2.17, 2.23-24)

Joseph Campbell, in his book *Pathways to Bliss*, explores the importance of following our calling in life based on the teachings of the Upanishads. He describes one of the pathways to enlightenment as 'following your bliss', writing:

> 'Your bliss can guide you to that transcendent mystery, because bliss is the welling up of the energy of the transcendent wisdom within you. So when the bliss cuts off, you know that you've cut off the welling up; try to find it again.' (Campbell, 2004)

The Hindu tradition talks about following your 'dharma', which is a Sanskrit word that means path or teaching. This has similarities to the Ancient Greek concept of eudaimonia and implies the true vocation set out for you. This 'welling up of the energy of the transcendent wisdom within you' seems similar to the concept of flow from positive psychology and also relates to the HCBT concept of spirit. The Bhagavad Gita is the Hindu text which portrays the following of this vocation or sacred duty. It tells the story of the warrior Arjuna who receives guidance from Krishna as to how to live out his dharma.

The concept of the Third Eye in Indian faith traditions may also have similarities to the concept of the spirit. The Third Eye relates to the chakra (an energy focal point in the body) called the Ajna on the brow between the eyes. This is seen as a gateway to higher realms of consciousness and ultimately to enlightenment and is believed to lead to visions and a deeper knowing and awareness. There are overlapping concepts found in various traditions of 'the mind's eye', 'the eyes of the heart' or the 'sixth sense', all of which point to a seeing that comes from the spirit rather than from our physical senses.

Buddhism and Taoism

Within the psychological world, Buddhism is probably best known for reminding the Western world of mindfulness, which we had largely lost contact with, though this practice can be found in all faith traditions in some form. Mindfulness helps us to still our minds in order to connect with our true centre, and the advancement of mindfulness in mental health has led to a revolutionary shift in well-being within Western society over the past few decades. Various images are used in mindfulness to suggest that there is a core part of us that is constant and stable as compared to passing emotions, thoughts and life experiences. These include the image of a mountain with passing weather and clouds going by, and the image of a river with passing fish or leaves floating by. In both images the mountain and the river remain constant.

In Buddhist texts, Buddha is quoted saying:

> 'Light the lamp within; strive hard to attain wisdom.' (The Dhammapada)

This inner lamp is called 'Anatta' in Buddhism, which actually means 'no-soul' and relates to the importance of detachment. This refers to the Buddhist idea that there are momentary selves that are not long lasting but are ever changing. Buddhism teaches that it is therefore important not to become too attached to any one of these identities.

However, Buddhism also teaches that we all have an essence which is a person's inherent nature and is made up of wisdom and compassion. Our essence gives us the capacity to be compassionate and to be at peace, which is the 'Buddha nature' within each person. Buddhists talk about the seed of Buddha being in every living thing. A key focus in Buddhism is developing our awareness of our Buddha nature and constantly evolving our consciousness. This can eventually lead to enlightenment or spiritual awakening. Thich Nhat Hanh is one of the world's leading Buddhist teachers and in his book *Silence* he says:

> 'Our mind is filled with noise, and that's why we can't hear the call of life, the call of love. Our heart is calling us, but we don't hear. We don't have the time to listen to our heart… Our true home is what the Buddha called the island of self, the peaceful place inside of us. Oftentimes we don't notice it's there; we don't even really know where we are, because our outer or inner environment is filled with noise. We need some quietness to find that island of self.' (Thich Nhat Hanh, 2015)

Within Buddhism, as well as some other Eastern traditions, is the idea of three minds or three centres of awareness – the head, heart and hara. The head is the centre of thinking intelligence and the source of consciousness; the heart is the centre of feeling intelligence; and the hara is the centre of bodily intelligence and gut feelings. Mindfulness, conscious breathing and other practices that develop awareness can be used to connect with these three centres of thinking, feeling and gut awareness. 'Hara' is a Japanese word for belly and it represents the centre of the soul, and could be related to the HCBT concept of spirit. Another related concept in Buddhism is 'shin', which means heart, core or true essence. An ancient Taoism saying is that:

> 'When you are sick, do not seek a cure. Find your centre and you will be healed.'

Spiritual but not Religious (SBNR)

The 'Spiritual But Not Religious' umbrella includes a wide range of beliefs and practices, some associated with the 'New Age' (Age of the Aquarius) such as animal spirits and guardian angels, as well as more feminist and eco-spiritualties and practices based on ancient Pagan traditions such as Wicca, Shamanism and Druidism. The fight to raise awareness about the fragility of the earth, and our need to care more for the natural world in which we live, is a way that many people are currently expressing their spirituality. This growth in awareness about issues of climate change has also prompted a growth in spirituality with beliefs about an interconnection with our spirits to the wider Spirit, Universe or Mother Nature.

Within Spiritual But Not Religious beliefs is often the belief of a divine power or energy that infuses the universe and humankind. Various names are given to this energy or sacred power such as Gaia or Mother Nature or the Universe, with the idea that the Universe works with us when we are moving in the right direction. So the concept of spirit within these spiritualties is something that connects us to the rest of humanity and to the wider eco-system. Various movements have developed, teaching that we are spiritual beings. For example, the 'Human Potential Movement' has developed humanistic beliefs and encourages the tapping into our full potential, and it holds that ultimately we are divine and should live from this place of divinity. Terms used within these spiritualties that may relate to the concept of spirit are 'droplet of divinity', 'inner Godhead' and 'divine self'.

Eckhart Tolle is a key spiritual leader in this field with his bestselling books *The Power of Now* and *A New Earth: Awakening to Your Life's Purpose*. He describes being overcome with anxiety and reaching a crisis point when he thought:

> '"I cannot live with myself any longer." This was the thought that kept repeating itself in my mind. Then suddenly I became aware of what a peculiar thought it was. "Am I one or two? If I cannot live with myself, there must be two of me: the 'I' and the 'self' that 'I' cannot live with." "Maybe", I thought, "only one of them is real".' (Tolle, 1997)

This began his journey into a new awareness of a deeper true self hidden beneath his anxious self. He describes a danger of over-identifying with the roles we play so that we begin to believe that our role is our identity. He encourages us to be in:

> '…that timeless state of intense conscious presence in the Now, so as to give you a taste of enlightenment… Moreover, since every person carries the seed of enlightenment within, I often address myself to the knower in you who dwells behind the thinker, the deeper self that immediately recognizes spiritual truth, resonates with it, and gains strength from it.' (Tolle, 1997)

He advocates, along with all the wisdom traditions, the importance of silence as the way to the spirit, as he says in his book *Stillness Speaks*:

> 'When you lose touch with inner stillness, you lose touch with yourself. When you lose touch with yourself, you lose yourself in the world. Your innermost sense of self, of who you are, is inseparable from stillness. This is the I Am that is deeper than name and form.' (Tolle, 2016)

The work of Abraham-Hicks and the ideas based on the law of attraction have also become increasingly popular in the West. They describe an inner Emotional Guidance System that has an emotional scale along which we can move up or down in a graded way. This scale can highlight whether or not we're connected to what they call 'the Source'.

Humanism

Humanistic psychology recognises a driving force within individuals towards self-actualisation and realising one's potential, which could relate to the HCBT concept of spirit.

Rogers (1951) described an innate tendency in people to grow towards positive change. He described how wholeness comes through understanding the unique self and learning to love and accept who we are. The basis of Rogerian, person-centred therapy, is that a person can reach their full potential and live according to their unique self if they are given the right conditions for such growth. Rogers identified these therapeutic core conditions of growth as being empathy, genuineness and unconditional positive regard. Within humanism there is also the idea that the human spirit is a collective force that brings us together in a shared humanity. This collective human spirit is working towards developing humanity as a whole.

Maslow's hierarchy of needs is a well-known stage model represented by a triangular diagram showing different levels of need, beginning with our basic needs for food and shelter at the bottom. As we move up the triangle the needs at the top are identified as our highest motivations for self-fulfilment and reaching one's full potential. Maslow's later versions of the model also added a final level at the apex, which was the need for transcendence; the need to be part of something bigger than ourselves and to experience the transpersonal. Maslow said:

> 'The spiritual life is part of our biological life. It is the highest part of it, but yet part of it. The spiritual life is part of the human essence. It is a defining characteristic of human nature, without which human nature is not full human nature. It is part of the real self, of one's identity, of one's inner core, or one's species-hood, of full humanness.' (Maslow, 1954)

Maslow described a latent greatness or higher level of consciousness that is in all of us and which can momentarily appear as 'peak experiences'. These are glimpses of what the self could be and the potential in all of us as part of our humanity. His studies focused on identifying the attributes of those people who reached self-actualisation; those who Maslow felt were being all that they could be and reaching their potential. He described self-actualisation as:

> 'Acceptance and expression of the inner core or self ie. actualisation of these latent capacities and potentialities, full functioning availability of the human and personal essence.' (Maslow, 1954)

He also had the idea of plateau living where the peak experience becomes the new way of living. He described this new state of being as:

> '…synonymous with selfhood, with being authenticated, with being a person, with being fully human.' (Maslow,1954)

So the spirit in humanistic terms is seen as fully part of the body and mind and not a separate part, which is linked to or made from the divine. It is therefore not seen as an entity that can live on after death. Within humanism, spirituality is viewed as part of being human, and connecting to something bigger than ourselves, is about connecting to each other and the world around us without needing to connect to a divine being. The spiritual life is therefore part of our everyday life and human existence. Professor

Richard Norman, a humanist philosopher, describes how the term 'spirit' can feel understandably uncomfortable for some atheists and humanists with its associations with spirituality and religious vocabulary. He defines the human spirit as:

> '…a shared vitality which enriches and inspires people and their lives and gives them a motivation to carry on with a sense of being part of some movement greater than themselves.' (Norman, 2018)

Within our humanity, the human spirit is seen to give meaning and purpose through living life to its full potential, through relationships and creativity, by making the world a better place in some way, and by putting something of ourselves into what we do. Seligman's work on signature strengths, within Positive Psychology, could be seen as helping to understand what is within our spirit and that our signature strengths and all that helps to make us flourish is coming from this place.

Analytical psychology

Jung suggested that we need to return to the ancient wisdom traditions in order to understand the spirit, which he described as:

> '…the life of the body, the life-breath, or a kind of life-force which assumed spatial and corporeal form at birth and left the dying body again after the final breath… Where do all our good and helpful flashes of intelligence come from? What is the source of our enthusiasms, inspirations and of our heightened feeling for life? The primitive senses in the depths of his soul the springs of life; he is deeply impressed with the life-dispensing activity of his soul.' (Jung, 1933)

In describing his therapeutic work, Jung said:

> 'The course of the physician is less a question of treatment than of developing the creative possibilities that lie in the patient himself… Each of us carries his own life-form – an indeterminable form which cannot be superseded by any other. About a third of my cases are suffering from no clinically definable neurosis, but from the senselessness and emptiness of their lives. It seems to me however that this can well be described as the general neurosis of our time.' (Jung, 1933)

Analytical psychology, based on Jung's work, encourages people to work towards self-realisation and individuation, which is about developing the potential of who they distinctively are. Jung spoke about his concerns of the reductionist views of psychodynamic therapy and scientific materialism and suggested that:

> '…we moderns are faced with the necessity of rediscovering the life of the spirit (the urge of life); we must experience it anew for ourselves. It is the only way in which we can break the spell that binds us to a cycle of biological events … that the human psyche from time immemorial has been shot through with religious feelings and ideas … and that the ego is ill for the very reason that it is cut off from the whole, and has lost its connection with mankind as well as the spirit… It is easy enough to drive the spirit out of the door, but when we have done so the salt of life goes flat.' (Jung, 1933)

He goes on to describe psychological difficulties as:

> '…the suffering of a human being who has not discovered what life means for him' and what will the therapist do when 'he sees only too clearly why his patient is ill; when he sees that it arises from his having no love, but only sexuality; no faith, because he is afraid to grope in the dark; no hope, because he is disillusioned by the world and by life; and no understanding, because he has failed to read the meaning of his own existence?' (Jung, 1933)

Within the process of individualisation, a person moves towards their own destiny and, as Jung said:

> '…individuality embraces our innermost, last, and incomparable uniqueness, it also implies becoming one's own self. We could therefore translate individuation as "coming to selfhood" or "self-realization".' (Jung, 1966)

Jungian psychologist Robert Johnson explains this individualisation process:

'Because this process of actualizing oneself and becoming more complete also reveals one's special, individual structure. It shows how the universal human traits and possibilities are combined in each individual in a way that is unlike anyone else.' (Johnson, 1991)

Jung spoke about two halves of life. The first half corresponds with the first stages of Maslow's triangle, and is about developing a healthy ego and focusing on external goals of building a career, relationships and an external identity and security. The second half of life, as described by Jung, is more about our inner life, uncovering aspects of the unconscious and integrating the shadow side of the personality so that we become more grounded, integrated human beings. In this second stage of life, meaning no longer comes so much from our external accomplishments but is from an internal source, which he termed the Self to distinguish it from the ego, and said:

> 'One cannot live the afternoon of life according to the programme of life's morning; for what was great in the morning will be of little importance in the evening, and what in the morning was true will at evening become a lie.' (Jung, 1966)

Third wave CBT

Some of the ideas from third wave CBT approaches have developed concepts that are similar to the HCBT concept of the spirit. For example, compassion-focused therapy (Gilbert, 2009) uses mindfulness to develop our 'compassionate mind' in order to be more compassionate to ourselves and others. In mindfulness-based CBT (Segal *et al*, 2002) and acceptance and commitment therapy (ACT), the concept of the 'observing self' (or 'self-in-context') is used to define the constant aspect of the person that is able to mindfully observe changing thoughts and feelings. Within dialectical behaviour therapy (DBT) there is the concept of the wise mind, which is defined by Linehan as:

> '…that part of each person that can know and experience truth. It is where the person knows something to be true or valid. It is almost always quiet, it has a certain peace. It is where the person knows something in a centred way.' (Linehan, 1993)

Within third wave CBT there is also a greater emphasis on the importance of values. For example, ACT encourages people to explore their values and to have more 'value-based behaviours' (Hayes *et al*, 1999).

Along with the importance of mindfulness and values, these concepts of the observing self, the compassionate mind and the wise mind seem to overlap to some degree with the concept of the spirit used within the HCBT model.

Transpersonal psychology

Within the psychology world, the human spirit is most directly explored within transpersonal psychology. This brings the perennial wisdom of spiritual traditions into the arena of psychology and recognises that there is a spiritual aspect to explore alongside the psychological. In transpersonal psychology there are a range of authors who explore the concepts of the Real, True or Transpersonal Self. These concepts generally have a common thread of reaching our potential, being authentic, developing in consciousness and recognising our wider interconnection with the spiritual and natural world around us. John Rowan described transpersonal approaches as those which:

> '…emphasize the spiritual centre in people; the direction of the person, the higher potentials of the person, the deeper perspective given by a sense of the divine … to do with the higher unconscious as distinct from the lower unconscious.' (Rowan, 2005)

Frances Clark describes an underlying assumption in transpersonal therapy is that:

> '…each human being has impulses toward spiritual growth, the capacity for growing and learning throughout life and that this growth can be facilitated and enhanced by psychotherapy … so that there is a shift from working on yourself to working with yourself.' (Clark, 1973)

She goes on to describe the process of learning to recognise and listen to the voice of inner wisdom or 'transpersonal self', which she defines as:

> '…that centre of pure awareness which simultaneously transcends and observes conflicts at the level of ego and personality … and gives a point of reference for the newly awakened sense of self. The continuing search for inner truth requires a sincere commitment to this transpersonal self and to begin to trust this inner intuition as we discern this inner voice above self-deceptions and distractions.' (Clark, 1973)

Similarly, the founder of biosynthesis, David Boadella, says:

> 'The task of all true therapies and the aim of the core teaching in all true religions is to re-connect us with the depth of ourselves … religion has used the God for the inexhaustible depth and ground of being… We need to help the person to find his inner ground, the source from which his own healing energy wells up with the power to integrate him anew.' (Boadella, 1987)

Roberto Assagioli (1965) developed a transpersonal approach called psychosynthesis. This therapeutic model encourages people to develop their sense of self, or 'I', by bringing together what might be in their lower unconsciousness (including such things as their shadow side, hidden drives and impulses) as well as their higher unconsciousness (including such things as strengths, creativity and their spiritual side) and 'synthesising' these different aspects to create a more coherent holistic identity. Psychosynthesis uses the terms 'Self' or 'Spirit' to represent a Transpersonal Self which directs and shapes the individual identity. Psychosynthesis uses the analogy that our thoughts, emotions and different aspects of our makeup are like instruments in the orchestra and the self is the conductor. Without a conductor directing the music, the orchestra can become disorganised with different competing sounds just producing noise. The conductor's role is to bring in the different sections and instruments as needed, and to combine them in order to make beautiful music. The conductor represents that central position of the spirit that helps to integrate the parts into a whole. Within this analogy psychosynthesis describes an unseen composer, the Transpersonal Self, who is the author of the music.

A key figure in transpersonal psychology who has studied the development of consciousness is Ken Wilber. He has researched in detail two hundred theories from diverse schools of thought, psychology models and spiritual traditions to develop his Integral Psychology. A key theme about personal development that is suggested in both psychosynthesis and in Wilber's work is the idea of the 'Great Nest of Being', as he describes it (Wilber, 2000). This is the principle that we don't lose former developmental stages as we progress, but they are incorporated within us and we build on each stage like small Russian dolls hidden within larger dolls.

Wilber describes how this Great Nest of Being starts with a conscious awareness of our bodies and a focus on physical objects, and then moves to an awareness of the mind, then to the soul, and then finally to the spirit at the highest level. He prefers to see these levels of consciousness as waves that merge into each other like colours of a rainbow which are more fluid than discrete levels. These developmental levels of consciousness are described as potentials that are in every one of us. We will not all move through each level so that, for some people, there will be levels that will always remain as potentials which are not realised. Wilber advocates for an integral psychology that spans the full range of human experience and explores different structures, functions and states of consciousness within each developmental stage. He uses the idea of four quadrants to include all aspects of life within integral psychology. These quadrants are the individual interior (our psychological and spiritual makeup); individual exterior (our physical body and behaviours); collective interior (relationships and culture) and collective exterior (our environment and social systems).

Wilber distinguishes between who we are externally, which he labels as the Observed self, and who we are internally, our Observing self. He describes how both these aspects of Observed and Observing self combine to give an overall sense of self. We have already suggested that the HCBT concept of spirit could relate to this idea of the Observing self when we discussed acceptance and commitment therapy (ACT) which also uses the concept of the Observing self. Wilber describes how our locus of identity moves more towards identifying with the internal Observing self rather than the external Observed self as we progress through the developmental stages.

Within Integral Psychology, the Observing self is seen as similar to the causal body in Hinduism, and is at the heart of who we are:

> '…the body of pure, unmoving consciousness – the Witness … that ever-present awareness is Spirit in us. That underlying current of constant consciousness (or nondual awareness) is a direct and unbroken ray of pure Spirit itself. It is our connection to God and Goddess, our pipeline straight to Source.' (Wilber *et al*, 2008)

So to conclude this journey through different faiths, philosophies and schools of psychology, it is interesting to see common threads and similar beliefs emerging across different times, different cultures and schools of thought. Despite the use of various terms and definitions relating to the concept of the spirit, there are many similarities. However, these concepts do not totally map onto each other and it is not the aim of HCBT to develop one definitive definition of the spirit but to value the richness of different perspectives.

Returning to the HCBT model, the small symbol of the spiral within the formulation represents this wealth of ideas and themes relating to the concept of our human spirit. The spiral was chosen intuitively to represent spirit and it was only a later discovery by the author that the spiral is an ancient symbol of spirituality and a symbol of the inner journey in various traditions. The spirit, as we discussed in the last chapter, is also represented by the image of the tree, which similarly has a rich symbolic history in various traditions.

Chapter 4: The HCBT developmental model

Now that we have explored the HCBT model and the concept of the spirit we will move on to look at the developmental aspect of the model. This model is based on various traditions and schools of thought, and as a developmental process could be described as a psycho-spiritual process. It draws from ideas that we explored in the proceeding chapter – from psychosynthesis, the work of Jung, Ignatian spirituality and other contemplative traditions, and the work of transpersonal psychologist Ken Wilber. It also draws on the concepts of False Self and True Self, which were mentioned in Thomas Merton's work in the last chapter and were introduced in psychology by Donald Winnicott in the 1960s (Winnicott, 1965). It builds on Waterman's ideas of combining an existential and essentialistic approach to how our identity is formed, which was mentioned at the beginning of Chapter 2. So, most of these ideas are not new, but they are not usually considered within a CBT framework. As with all these models, it is not prescriptive but suggests a possible model of development, knowing that in reality how we develop is far more complex. As you will see, this developmental model of self still fits within the HCBT model and we will link it back to the Free to be Me course at the end of this chapter.

Stages of development

In Chapter 2 we used the analogy of a multi-coloured glass lantern to represent different aspects of personhood. It will be helpful to keep this image in mind as we explore the developmental model of HCBT (Figure 4.1: Lantern). In this developmental process we will see that our focus of attention moves through the three main aspects of our being – physical, psychological and spiritual.

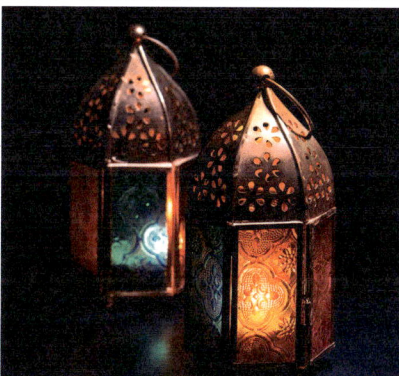

Figure 4.1: Lantern

As we have already said, the frame of the lantern represents the body and this gives the external shape and form of the individual. If we consider the process of development, when a baby is born their focus is on their physical needs – food, sleep and warmth. Babies are fascinated by what they experience through their senses; looking and listening and also tasting everything they can. They are discovering their hands and feet and what they can do, and gradually learning what is good to chew on and what isn't so good. As they develop and learn, they begin to recognise the boundary of their own body in relation to others and they learn that they are a separate individual from their caregivers. So, the first developmental stage is on the discovery of who they are physically and how they look, and to some degree this will continue into the next phase too. Their body's senses help them to understand the world around them and they begin to form thoughts and ideas based on their life experiences. This leads to the next focus of attention in their development: the psychological aspect.

Here, their focus is on developing their sense of an external self. This concept of external self relates to the psychodynamic term of ego or persona and this developmental phase matches with Jung's first stage of his individuation process which we looked at in the previous chapter. Their external self is the life they create for themselves and how they define themselves, and is the psychological identity that they show to the world. It includes what defines them in terms of their chosen preferences, the skills they learn, their career choices, what they choose to own and invest their time and money in and the relationships they form. Some of what they develop at this stage may be in response to external pressures, coming from other people's expectations and imposed goals for their lives. Other aspects of their external self may develop as a reaction to life's experiences, whether negative or positive. This phase also includes the physical focus of the first stage, and so their body image, their looks and how they are seen are also part of this external self.

As we said in Chapter 2, the glass of the lantern represents a person's psychological make up and their external self is represented by the range of glass used. The different pieces of glass in the lantern are made up of a variety of colours and shapes, which represents their individuality and the richness of each of us as a unique person. The person's external self can be seen as being made up of a range of selves and different aspects of their external self are more dominant in different settings and in different relationships. They have many different sides to their sense of self, which are likely to change over time as well as across different situations. So, for example, staying with our lantern analogy, the colours they show at work may be different to what their partner sees when they get home. They can experiment with different colours and shapes of glass but gradually over time they will build a sense of self that, depending on their life experiences and psychological well-being, becomes a relatively stable sense of self. This develops like the glass sides of the lantern within the frame and aspects of these colours are seen by those around them.

Another way of seeing this process comes from narrative psychology and is the idea that we are writing a particular story about ourselves, that we tell to ourselves and to others. This story of our identity or external self is something we weave from the different life events and experiences we have. However, we have a selective memory and our stories can be based on our own perceptions, biases and beliefs. This means that our version of our story may not always fit with other people's perceptions of us. Our story can be more about how we perceive ourselves or maybe how we wish to be perceived by others, rather than how others actually perceive us.

The final aspect of this developmental model is the focus on the spirit, which is represented by the lit candle at the heart of the lantern. This is the spiritual part of our identity. We have already explored the concept of the spirit in Chapter 3 and have seen that there are different ways people relate to the concept of the spirit and different spiritualties. This final stage of development is therefore about connecting more with this inner spirit or deeper self and living an authentic life, responding from this place of spirit. This is the stage of questioning what life is all about and thinking more about finding meaning and identifying purpose in life beyond the developing of the external self. As with other previous stages, the third stage encapsulates the previous stages and so incorporates who a person is physically and psychologically, to form a more holistic and centred sense of self. The final focus is therefore the development of a spiritual identity that helps to enliven and strengthen the psychological and physical aspects already developed. (This is similar to the second stage in Jung's individuation process.) This process of change towards more existential questions can feel uneasy and shaky and so some people may retreat back into building their external self rather than having the courage to let go of aspects of more unhealthy versions of self. This may be what partly drives the stereotypical midlife crisis of buying expensive cars or experimenting with new beauty treatments. These strengthen the external, and possibly unhealthier, versions of self, in the face of passing years, in order to avoid the more existential questions bubbling up from within.

To summarise these stages, once a person has gained a sense of physical identity as a young child, they then begin to build their external psychological and physical self; forming relationships, developing interests which may later lead to building a career, buying possessions and creating a certain life they choose and develop. In this earlier stage their sense of worth often comes from what they do, who they mix with and what they own. However, there sometimes comes a time, perhaps later in life, when they begin to question whether this is all life has to offer and they may start to focus more on questions of meaning and purpose; more existential questions that take them deeper, beyond the externals of life. Their sense of self in this phase comes more from who they are as much as, or even more than, what they do; their focus is more on developing their character and authenticity.

Developing healthier versions of self

Thinking again about the HCBT formulation and the helpful and unhelpful cycles, the more a person moves towards helpful patterns of thoughts and behaviours, the more they are developing an external self that is in line with the spirit. This external self, based on helpful cycles, will then lead to the development of healthier versions of themselves. Depending on the external self that a person has developed, their spirit can be hidden to a greater or lesser extent. As Oprah Winfrey has been quoted saying, 'We don't hide our secrets, our secrets hide us'.

Some aspects of a person's external self may have developed as a reaction to life events and contextual influences, and therefore these aspects will not feel in tune or in line with their spirit; the external self does not resonate with their spirit. When their external self is in conflict with their spirit then we could say that those aspects of their external self are developing more unhealthy versions of their self. Within our analogy of the lantern, this could be described as darkened glass within the lantern which stops the spirit's light shining through. It doesn't destroy the spirit, the flame is always there, but the unhealthier versions of their self can hide it and limit who they truly are.

In contrast, there may be aspects of their external self which is more like opaque glass. It still has their individual colours but allows more of that internal flame to shine through which accentuates the external self to make the colours look richer and more alive. When the external self is in line with their spirit then the light can shine more brightly through those colours of glass and if they are fully integrated externally with who they are internally, this leads to healthier versions of self being developed. So, this is not to say that all our external selves are false, unhealthy or need letting go – but it is a process of discerning what is helpful and authentic and what is disconnected from our spirit. These healthier versions of self develop from the spirit and the spirit literally acts as a 'spirit level' or benchmark for this process. The healthier version of a person is achieved when the person is integrated inside and out, having a sense of who they are within, as well as what they have built up externally. Their external self is also stronger because of that connection to what is within.

There are no ages attached to these phases of growth within the HCBT model. Many primary aged children are quite authentic and integrated with healthy versions of self, though they may not be able to reflect on these experiences or learn from them as they will do later in life. As they grow there is a danger that they can become distanced from who they truly are as education and family potentially shapes them and redirects their focus. The 'second half of life' – focusing more on developing their healthy, authentic self – can come at any age and there are often sparks of it throughout a person's life. The challenge is for each of us to recognise these inner sparks and give them permission to shape who we are; learning 'to live from the centre'.

This is something to consider for those of us who are parents or educators – are we encouraging young people to recognise what is authentically them and what is part of the heathier versions of self rather than imposing our expectations on them, which may not fit with who they naturally are? Are we allowing them to try what they are instinctively drawn to and resonate with rather than trying to shape them a certain way? Depending on the parenting, the opportunities a child is given and the ongoing encouragement they have to develop healthier versions of self, there is the possibility that a person could develop holistically and authentically with the 'two halves of life' happening in parallel. So, though we talk about the first half and the second half of life, these two stages could happen together; growing both an external self and also discovering the inner self in order to develop healthier versions of self as an authentic whole.

We could potentially have a developmental process of stages in which a person first develops their external self and then they begin to question and review this external self that they have built up. Ideally, this person will learn to listen to their spirit and to recognise healthier versions of self in order to learn what resonates within their deeper selves. They can then use this process of recognition as a benchmark to gradually review what they have built up as their external self. Over time they have the potential to chip away some of the pieces that no longer sit well within their frame and replace it with pieces which feel more aligned to who they are. As the famous sculptor Michelangelo is reported to have said when asked how he created his statue of David, 'It is easy. You just chip away the stone that doesn't look like David.' However there may be some aspects of the external self which are already in line with the person's spirit and so instead of chipping these away, they need strengthening and developing.

Going back to the analogy of storytelling, the process of developing more healthy versions of ourselves could be seen as reflecting on the story we have written so far and editing and refining it, even rewriting it where needed. It is changing and developing it and potentially discovering a new story for our lives, a story that may go in a different direction to the trajectory that we might have assumed for ourselves. This developmental process of self-discovery is often portrayed in myths and fairy stories in which the hero overcomes various battles and trials to discover their true potential or hidden identity.

In order to reach this state of total integration there is often a letting go of parts that a person may quite like, parts of their unhealthy self that they have become attached to as aspects of themselves. Within the various wisdom traditions is the challenge of 'dying to self', or becoming 'detached' in order to become who we truly are. In the process of becoming a fully integrated person there is this process of 'dying to' or 'detaching' from unhealthier versions of our external self. This is a process of letting go of what was never truly them in the first place; letting go of what they thought they were to become who they truly are which is always better and more authentic than unhealthier versions of self. However, they can only let go of aspects of their unhealthy self if they know what these aspects are. A person therefore needs a certain level of a 'sense of self' in order to begin to question the self and to allow it to be shaped and pruned. We need to have some degree of 'knowing thyself' before we can start trying to 'die to self'. Both of these processes are lifelong and are often haphazard stages which involve experimenting with different interests, relationships and ways of being to find what resonates and fits with who we truly are. It is also a lifelong process of thinking that we know who we truly are, only to discover that this is another layer of an unhealthy version of self that needs pruning and refining. It often needs trusted relationships around us and time to reflect on this process to keep learning and maturing.

If we relate these ideas back to the HCBT formulation, we can see that when a person is responding in helpful cycles, their spirit is freer and they are responding from this place and so creating healthier versions of self. Alternatively, when they are reacting in unhelpful cycles then they are creating and strengthening unhealthier versions of their self which don't fit with their inner spirit and are not authentic. For example, a person may move between an unhealthy, anxious version of themselves and a healthy more self-confident version of themselves. By detaching from these unhelpful anxious cycles, they can let go of the more unhealthy versions of themselves and move to the more helpful, confident cycles in order to develop healthier versions of self.

If we think of this process in psychodynamic terms, the more disturbed their early attachment relationship has been to their caregivers, the more a person's external self will be made up of defences. This unhealthy external self can be improved as the person learns to recognise these defences and connects more with their spirit and true self.

Connecting to the wider context

As we have discussed earlier in this book, we do not live in a vacuum and it is important to see ourselves within a wider context. This is also true within this developmental model.

At each stage of this developmental process a person's context has a huge impact on them – from being young children who are totally dependent on those around them, to the next stages of development where they are forming their identity in relation to others and creating a life for themselves among the wider world in which they find themselves. In the more spiritual stages of development where the focus is on developing an authentic self, it is difficult to have a sense of wholeness if a person sees themselves in a vacuum. So rather than focusing just on developing a person in isolation, this journey may move towards recognising themselves as one piece of a cosmic jigsaw. This shift in perspective can on one level make us feel very small in comparison to such a vast backdrop. However, on another level it also heightens the value of each person as an individual with importance, and all of us being needed to build an interconnected whole. As well as letting go of aspects of their unhealthy versions of self and developing more authentic aspects of who they are, a person may also recognise their interconnectedness at a deeper level. There is therefore the need for each of us to develop who we truly are, not just for ourselves but for each other so that we might fit more comfortably alongside others into the universal whole. Again, this idea is found in the wisdom traditions in which there is the belief of a spiritual awareness that recognises something that was always present; that we are part of something bigger than ourselves, whether that is in terms of being part of a wider ecosystem, a network of relationships or being connected to, or part of, the divine or the Universe. In the HCBT model, we sometimes refer to this as Life's Source and Flow.

Maslow's work on self-actualisers found a similar awareness of being part of a wider context, of people having a cause they believed in or a vocation they were devoted to. This led self-actualisers to be altruistic and:

> '… involved in a cause outside their own skin, in something outside of themselves.' (Maslow, 1954)

The importance of looking beyond ourselves, not only for the good of others but also for our own well-being, has been supported by research in positive psychology. This shows that looking outside of ourselves and focusing on others and on how we can help others is one of the main ways we boost our own well-being. As Seligman has said:

> 'We scientists have found that doing a kindness produces the single most reliable momentary increase in well-being of any exercise we have tested.' (Seligman, 2011)

So this developmental model is holistic in terms of the growing awareness of the interconnectedness of the physical, psychological and spiritual aspects within our identity. However, it is also holistic in the recognition that each of us, as individuals, are also interconnected with each other and with the world in which we live, and that to be healthy we need to be looking outwards as well as inwards.

Roles within our External self

We have talked about the external self in quite general terms, but let's now focus on the idea of roles which may help us to identify what we mean by the external self more clearly. This draws from the work of Roberto Assagioli who developed psychosynthesis and his ideas of sub-personalities (Assagioli, 1965). He suggests that we develop a number of fairly stable sub-personalities that may or may not be helpful. Psychosynthesis is about recognising and integrating these different personalities into a stable whole and has been described as a process of 'learning to live with the vision which comes from within yourself'. Within the HCBT model the spirit is at the heart of who we are and the place from where that vision of ourselves comes from.

Considering helpful and unhelpful HCBT cycles, a person can find themselves developing cycles of thoughts and behaviours which become consistent patterns of being. These stable ways of being then lead to the development of certain roles, for example, playing the role of the victim, the 'people pleaser', the bully or the clown. These default patterns of thoughts and behaviour, which form their roles, are often a response to whatever life has thrown at them. In reality a person does not just have one external self, but instead has a range of roles with which they identify. They can become any one of these roles according to different situations and together this collection of roles can form their external self. If these roles develop from within and are in line with their spirit then they can be helpful and feel healthy. However, if they are developed more as a reaction to painful events and are more defensive, they can make up unhealthier versions of their self. If they live within roles which are not true to who they are, they can sometimes find themselves getting burnout because they are having to work extra hard to do something which doesn't come naturally to them. Alternatively, they may find these roles unsatisfying so they can feel empty or bored with life because it doesn't really connect with what energises them.

We can now imagine each of these helpful and unhelpful cycles developing into a role. If we take this image one step further, then each of these roles are cycling round a central spirit, or core identity. We could picture this spirit being like a sun, which is stable at the core of a person's being and they have different roles that are like circling planets around this stable centre. At any one time their locus of identity can move from one role to another and they can express themselves in different ways.

For each of a person's roles we can draw helpful and unhelpful cycles showing the emotions, thoughts and behaviours associated with these roles. We can see that they have developed certain roles and that they move between them. We may find that some roles act as a balance to each other and may reflect opposing ways of being, for example an extrovert balancing an introvert role or a hard working role balancing out a more laid back playful role. We might find, in different stages of life or different situations, that different roles can take the lead. However, the other roles might still be there in the background or they might change or morph into new roles over time.

It may be helpful at this point to give an example of roles from some work carried out with a middle-aged, white British woman who identified four main roles. Firstly, there was the 'strict controller', which was quite a dominating and controlling role. This role helped her to get things done but could also be critical of herself and others. The unhelpful cycle underlying this role included emotions of stress and frustration, and her related thoughts included 'You have to do this right', 'This isn't good enough' and 'Hurry up'. Secondly, there was the 'motherly octopus', who was friendly and cheerful and worked hard at making sure everyone felt supported and everything was working well. This was a role which energised her and where she felt a sense of flow, which suggests this connected with her spirit. However, there was also a less healthy aspect of this role – that of a 'people pleaser', of worrying about what people thought and working excessively to get approval. Thirdly, there was the 'independent scholar' who enjoyed hiding away with a book and enjoying her own company, which again had healthy and unhealthy aspects: enjoying learning on one side, but withdrawing from others on the other. Finally, there was the 'sulky child'. This was another unhealthy role in which she thought herself to be unwanted and worried about being rejected. Identifying these four predominant roles helped in then identifying the related unhelpful and helpful cycles associated with each of these roles. By doing this, the person was able to be more aware of healthier versions of herself and move to more helpful cycles of thoughts and behaviours.

An awareness exercise that was developed in psychosynthesis and which has since emerged in the ACT literature is the meditation of the observing self. In this exercise, we are asked to be aware of our thoughts but recognise that we are not our thoughts, to be aware of our body but to recognise that we are not our body and so on. This exercise can also be done by reflecting on our different roles, recognising that we are observing our roles so we are therefore not our roles.

Over time, a person may begin to question their roles and ideally start to measure them up against the spirit; what resonates with who they truly are and what feels authentic? What in these roles is limiting their spirit and what is freeing it? What do they find helpful and want to keep, and what do they need to let go of? So the spirit acts as a spirit level, a central core and benchmark with which a person can reflect on these aspects of their external self.

The theory is that the more a person is in touch with their spirit the more they can be centred. From this centred place of the observing self they can then look objectively at these roles and develop their healthier identity from them. Alternatively, the more that their identity is enmeshed in one or two roles, the more they will tend to see themselves and the world around them through that lens. In this state they are less able to be objective about these roles and so are unable to develop a healthier identity from them. A healthier version of self develops as a widening circle from a person's spirit, at their centre, as they integrate helpful aspects of these roles which are in line with their spirit and which express who they truly are. This authentic healthy version of self is made up of a unique combination of the different roles that make up their personality but is grounded by the centre, their spirit.

In moving to a greater integration between internal and external identities, a person may need to let go of some of these roles. We can sometimes get attached to how people perceive us and we can have relationships and situations in our lives that are built on the roles that we have developed. There can therefore be a lot invested in maintaining these roles in order to maintain the status quo. If a person starts to question the roles and position they have formed for themselves, those around them may undermine their attempts to change. Their workplace, for example, may suit a certain role that they have been playing for years, which may serve a company well. They, too, may find it hard to let go of roles or to reshape them, and so this process may involve making choices and testing out changes in a gradual way. A person may hold on to the unhealthier versions of self, fearful of letting go of all that they have built up, and sometimes it's only when external life events occur such as a bereavement or redundancy that they are forced to revaluate the unhealthier versions of themselves. These crisis points can be the beginning of a letting go of these unhealthy versions and building a more healthy self and the opportunity for post traumatic growth.

HCBT and other developmental models

The work of Jung and his process of individuation and the influence of Assagioli's psychosynthesis have already been referred to in relation to this HCBT developmental model. However, this developmental process is also reflected in Maslow's triangle of needs which starts with the physical needs of food and shelter and then moves through the layers of psychological needs such as self-esteem, belonging and aesthetic needs, and up to the levels of spiritual needs of meaning, transcendence and interconnectedness. Maslow described the ongoing process of becoming self-actualised as being based on the choices we make:

> 'Let us think of life as a process of choices, one after another. At each point there is a progression choice and a regression choice. There may be a movement toward defence, toward safety, toward being afraid; but over on the other side, there is the growth choice. To make the growth

choice instead of the fear choice a dozen times a day is to move a dozen times a day toward self-actualization… There is a self, and what I have sometimes referred to as "listening to the impulse voices" means letting the self emerge… One cannot choose wisely for a life unless he dares to listen to himself, his own self, at each moment in life.' (Maslow, 1971)

These developmental stages of HCBT are also seen in Ken Wilber's work in which he describes the focus of identity as being like the centre of gravity moving progressively from the body to the soul and then to the spirit. As mentioned in Chapter 3, Wilber developed the idea of different developmental levels within a 'Great Nest of Being'. For those familiar with his work, it may be helpful to describe the HCBT developmental process in terms of Wilber's model. Wilber's 'mental ego' level is similar to the formation of the external self. Wilber describes this as the most common and everyday level of consciousness. Ideally, we progress from this stage to Wilber's 'centaur level', which is characterised by autonomy and integration. This is the stage of questioning the roles and identity developed in the mental ego level and becoming more autonomous, integrated and authentic in discovering who we are, developing our true self.

John Rowan describes this development as going from:

'…the realm of deficiency (where all the motivation is to repair some deficit) to the realm of abundance (where the motivation comes from a positive urge to explore, create and grow) and it is about moving from a focus on having and doing to being.' (Rowan, 2005)

Beyond the centaur stage in Wilber's model is the 'subtle' or 'transpersonal' level. Wilber suggests that progression to this level helps to move us away from being too focused on our own individualised self-development and to recognise that we are part of a greater interconnectedness. The subtle level is about connecting with something bigger than ourselves and recognising an interconnectedness with others, and as a result there is a growth of awareness of others and of compassion. Wilber describes this stage as being the realm of the transpersonal, of paradoxes and mystery, of symbols and the sacred.

The HCBT developmental model within the Free to be Me course

Returning to the HCBT formulation, we can see that we have two cycles – the unhelpful and helpful cycles of thoughts, emotions and behaviour along with physical sensations. These then lead to both short-term and long-term consequences. The consequences, as we have seen in this chapter, are that by continuing to act a certain way over time, a person's patterns of behaviour can develop into relatively stable identities and roles.

The unhelpful cycles will go on to form aspects of unhealthy versions of self which can become fixed unhelpful patterns of thinking and behaviour that limit the person's spirit and so limit their connection and development of healthier versions of self. In the helpful cycles, by contrast, they are developing healthy aspects of their external self which are in line with their spirit and so help them to develop and strengthen a healthier version of self.

Thinking about the HCBT model, by connecting more with that internal spirit they can find the resources to make changes to build a healthier external self which is more aligned to the blueprint of their spirit. The two cycles in the formulation represent the choice which a person has at any one time to move closer to being a healthier form of self or further away from it. Our healthy self represents the highest form of who we can be and each life decision, large or small, can move us nearer to releasing that potential, or move us further away. In some situations, we may have choices that are equally healthy or equally unhealthy, but as Maslow described, in any given moment we have two options: to step forward into growth or to step back into fear, and those who self-actualise are those stepping forward.

The Free to be Me course aims to help people to recognise these unhelpful and helpful cycles and also to recognise and develop aspects of their external self that are in line with their healthier self. Participants of the Free to be Me course will be at different stages of this developmental journey. The majority are likely to be still building and developing their external self and often they are doing so according to society's expectations, what others think of them and the roles they have developed so far. The HCBT model therefore provides an opportunity to do this development in a more conscious, authentic way so that they build and refine their external self in a way that resonates with their inner spirit. At this stage, HCBT is about helping people to develop a relatively stable self-image through identifying their strengths and the healthy roles within their life which gives them a sense of self-worth and value.

However, some course participants may have already developed a stable and healthy view of themselves, and for these participants the course may instead be the beginning of a life review. The journey may involve more reflecting on what has already been built and a letting go of some aspects of who they thought they were. This process of reviewing may have been kickstarted by life events that have challenged their previous self-concept, such as an unexpected bereavement or job loss that has made them question their values and identity. This is the stage of questioning their roles and identity that they have already developed and becoming more autonomous, integrated and authentic in who they are and 'being free to be me'. The title of the course has sometimes drawn people to the course in recognition that this is the journey they are already on and they resonate with the idea of being 'free to be me'.

Within this more psycho-spiritual journey, some participants may also have a sense of the transpersonal, and part of this journey of self-development might be the recognition that they are part of a greater interconnectedness. This can often lead to a more inclusive way of seeing others and greater compassion both for others, themselves and the world around them.

Chapter 5: HCBT as an individual therapy

Developing the HCBT formulation and drawing the tree to represent the idea of spirit initially grew out of individual therapy. These ideas were used to enrich our HCBT work and to include the client's views of themselves as a whole, particularly exploring their strengths and hopes. The therapy also gave more focus to the person's wider context, such as the influence of culture, family and their housing environment as well as giving space to talk about spirituality and how this inter-related with their presenting difficulties. So, although the HCBT model forms the basis of a group programme, its roots are within individual therapy and it can be used in this way.

As a therapist you may wish to pick out exercises or ideas from the *Free to be Me manual* to integrate into your existing therapeutic approach. However, if you wish to use the HCBT model and HCBT process in a more systematic way and follow the same journey as the Free to be Me course, then this chapter will give you an outline of how you may achieve this as individual therapy. Obviously, this approach loses the value of group dynamics and discussions, and the client doesn't have the peer support and sense of community which a group creates, but the advantages are that the therapy can be more tailored to the client's specific needs and allows more space to talk about personal issues. For clients who cannot speak English and so are not able to attend an English speaking Free to be Me group, this approach enables a client to benefit from the HCBT approach because the therapy can be offered with an interpreter. (However, the use of interpreters could also be considered within the Free to be Me group.)

Assessment

The first contact with a client is crucial for setting the foundations for the rest of the work. As with any therapy, the focus at assessment therefore needs to be about creating a trusting relationship by offering the client a space which feels safe and containing. The assessment session needs to allow the person time to talk about the issues they want to address in therapy and for them to feel heard and understood. This can be achieved through basic counselling skills such as active listening and accurate summaries to ensure that you understand what they are experiencing and get a sense of what it is like living in their shoes.

The assessment application form in the Free to be Me manual (Handout 0.1) can be used to gain basic information and contact details and is best done by asking the client to complete the first page and then using the questions on the second page as part of the assessment in a more conversational approach. It is also useful to ask the client to complete the outcome measures used for the group which are the PHQ-9, GAD-7 and SWEMWBS. Their answers to these could then be used to initiate questions about their mood and general well-being[1].

During this first assessment session you also need to check that you are the right person to work with this client and that this approach is suitable for them. For example, it is important to explore their level of risk, whether their difficulties are something you have the skills to work with, and whether they are ready to start the work. It is therefore useful to cover the following issues within the assessment:

- Have they just had, or are about to have, any major life events such as moving house, having a baby or being recently bereaved, which might suggest that this is not the right time to begin this work? Check if there are any issues that might hinder them from attending such as caring responsibilities or health issues.

- Do they use drugs and/or excessive use of alcohol? Therapy can trigger painful emotions or memories and so if people have used substances to cope in the past then there is a risk they may relapse or use excessively. Their dependency will need to be addressed first or in parallel to the therapy.

- How are their English skills? The course has quite a few handouts and written exercises so a basic level of literacy is ideal. In individual therapy, written material can be explained and simplified although it is still obviously easier if clients have basic skills in this area. If someone's first language is not English, you may wish to use an interpreter and the client can write in their own language.

- How motivated are they to attend weekly and to make changes? Clients need to be willing to engage in the process and to commit to attending regularly and with an open mind to try new things. The full course is 16 weeks but working individually allows you to tailor the sessions to the client's own needs and to adapt the course's length and contents.

- Are there any risk issues towards themselves or to others? Do they have any current thoughts of suicide, any self-harm or past suicide attempts and any potential safeguarding issues such as their behaviour towards children or vulnerable adults? If this is the case, you would need to decide if your level of skills and your setting enables you to safely manage this

---

1   To use the SWEMWBS measure you need to register for free, completing an online form at https://warwick.ac.uk/fac/sci/med/research/platform/wemwbs/using but the other two measures are available to use online.

risk or whether the person needs more immediate crisis work or referring elsewhere before doing this course.

- Have they had previous therapy and what was helpful and unhelpful from this? How would this course compare and what are their expectations of the course? These are useful areas to explore in the assessment session to gain a better understanding of any preconceived ideas or expectations that a client is coming with.

- Are there any other difficulties that you need to consider which may make this course inappropriate for this person, such as active psychotic symptoms or learning disabilities? Again, this depends on your level of skill and your setting and whether you are able to adapt the material for the people with whom you work.

Once the assessment is completed the final part of this meeting should include booking the date for the first session, assuming that the client is willing to engage with the therapy process.

Session outlines

The individual session outlines can be found at the end of each group session within the *Free to be Me manual*. Each individual session outline states the session's aims, content and the handouts needed. As well as the group handouts, each session has an individual handout that summarises the PowerPoint slides used in the group so that you do not need to use PowerPoint presentations in the individual sessions. However, you may wish to print off the group PowerPoint slides for your own reference.

As with the group process, it is important that you familiarise yourself with the material before the session and print off the handouts for the client. You may find it useful to also print a set of handouts for yourself to make it easier to explain them to the client. It is recommended that you adapt and individualise these session summaries to the client's own situation and difficulties. You may find it helpful to print off the relevant manual page before the session and to highlight key points from the group script that are relevant to use for the client. Working with an individual allows you to personalise the material even more than for a group, and in particular to adapt the terminology to align it with the client's own. You may prefer to follow the manualised approach the first few times you work individually with clients in order to familiarise yourself with the material, but in time you may find yourself creating your own style to the HCBT approach. In the group version of Free to be Me, someone may ask something that relates to a later session or a future exercise, and so the facilitator will explain that this will be covered later in the course. However, in individual sessions you have the freedom to jump around the course more freely, so that you could decide to swap the order of sessions or use an exercise from a later session at an earlier point if this would help the therapeutic process for your particular client.

The timing of group sessions is 2 hours long with a break, but for an individual session you would want to aim to make the session nearer to the usual therapy hour. This can be mutually agreed and you may find that some clients wish to do the activities within the session so you may choose to make sessions longer to accommodate this. Other clients may prefer to do these exercises in their own time and to bring them back to discuss the following week.

Each individual session should begin with a review of their week to allow some time to hear about any difficulties or issues which have arisen, but this need only take about 5–10 minutes so that the session does not turn into a general counselling session. Any exercises or goals that were planned from the week before can be discussed at the beginning of the session. Any obstacles in completing these exercises should be explored to consider ways to help the person complete the exercises, particularly those ones which seem most relevant to them.

The aims of the session should be briefly explained and then the session can include the suggested areas of discussion and activities from the group session outline, though you may prefer to change the order or omit certain activities depending on the client's needs. The other advantage of working individually is being able to adapt the content so that you can use the medium which best suits your client. For example, some people prefer to talk about issues whereas other clients may prefer to use art or reflective writing to engage with the material. HCBT can be done through ecotherapy sessions of walking in nature or through online video calls. Working individually gives you the freedom to explore how the client wishes to work with the material, while still following the HCBT model and basic course structure.

As with the group sessions, it is helpful for you to recognise your own journey with this material and it is advisable to have done the exercises yourself before you ask clients to complete them. Although you are not going to run the therapy as a group programme, it may still be useful for you to read the first few chapters of the manual on the process of HCBT and the practicalities of running the group so that you have a good understanding of the material.

The journal is an important part of the course because it encourages a growth in personal reflection and helps people to discern what resonates with them and what they are reacting to, which can lead to useful insights. The client may wish to write their journal at home, although if this is the case it is useful to check every now and again that they are completing this reflective process. Alternatively, time can be given to the journal writing at the end of each session and you may wish to leave the client to write on their own in the therapy room before coming back after a certain time to say goodbye, depending on your client and your therapy environment. Alternatively, you might both wish to sit and write an individual journal at the end of each session, and this offers you an alternative way of writing therapy case notes.

The final session should include time to reflect on the process as a whole and the client may choose to read through their journal before this session as a way of reflecting on the therapy journey. The final session should also revisit goals that they began therapy with as well as any goals that they have set along the way, and to think about how they will continue to work on these in the future. As with the group programme it can also be helpful to suggest any further support or services that may be beneficial for them as a next step or in case they need help in the future.

As well as growing out of individual work, HCBT grew out of a response to CBT being over manualised in some situations to the point of it becoming quite limited. If CBT is offered in an over manualised way then it loses the individualistic approach and the importance of building a therapeutic relationship in which the person's individual needs, context, background and world view are valued. This leads to the situation in which each person is offered the same basic format and techniques. So it is important to recognise that although the manual offers individual outlines for each session, these should be used as general guidelines and shaped according to the clients with whom you are working. The session outlines are to be used as guidance of general direction rather than step-by-step tasks that have to be followed rigorously. The focus always needs to be the client and their own personal development and this should decide what is done rather than trying to cover everything in each session.

Fatima: a case study of individual HCBT

The following case study is based on some work that was done when HCBT was still emerging as part of the individual work I was doing within the NHS. The client's name and some of the personal details have been changed to maintain her anonymity.

Fatima was from the Congo and was in her 30s. She lived with her three boys, who were all attending the same primary school. She was seen in an NHS mental health trust setting following a hospital admission, in which she had been diagnosed with psychosis. When the therapy started she was no longer presenting with severe psychotic symptoms though she still heard voices occasionally when she couldn't sleep. Her main presentation was of extreme anxiety and underlying PTSD symptoms.

She talked about memories of the war in her country and the atrocities she had witnessed, including the death of both her parents within a few years of each other. She was an orphan by the time she was 10 years old and was taken in by her aunt and uncle along with their six children. She described how she was used by the uncle's family as a servant and she was no longer allowed to attend school. Her uncle started to sexually abuse her when she turned 12, and this continued until she was helped by a neighbour to flee to the UK at age 19. During her escape she met another refugee with whom she had a relationship for about 10 years. They moved together to London but he had become increasingly abusive towards her and with the help of a women's refuge she had escaped this relationship. When I saw her, she was a single mother of three boys living in a high-rise council flat with two bedrooms, which was temporary accommodation.

The therapy work began with some standard trauma-focused CBT work which was used to reduce her flashbacks and other PTSD symptoms. This trauma work included the life map exercise which is now the main part of session 11 of the Free to be Me course. Related to her PTSD was her anxiety about going out and in particular her worry when her children had to go out. She found it especially difficult to take them to school and to trust that they would be safe there. The focus of the work that we then started to do was on developing her strength of identity and purpose. She was someone who recognised that she had a strong core of resilience and hope despite, or perhaps because of, her traumatic past. She recognised how far she had come in her journey of survival and the concept of post traumatic growth really resonated with her. Her main focus and purpose in life were her three boys and she wanted to offer them a secure home and to provide them with a good start in life. This gave her the motivation to face going out more. She initially did this more for her children but increasingly also for herself.

Figure 5.1: Case study formulation shows Fatima's personalised HCBT formulation. In individual therapy these tend to be handwritten and ideally use colours to highlight the helpful and unhelpful aspects of the formulation. Ideally, it is better if the client is able to write these themselves, with the therapist offering the template and guidance as to how to complete it. In particular, we used the helpful and unhelpful cycles at the bottom of the formulation for Fatima to recognise these patterns and to choose to move in more helpful cycles.

The therapy talked through the different aspects of this formulation and by focusing on the helpful as well as unhelpful cycles, Fatima became more conscious of the choices she was making in what was strengthening her sense of self and what was limiting this.

The formulation also enabled her to recognise the external influences around her more. The environmental influence was particularly significant and we discussed how living in a small, high-rise flat with three young boys impacted her well-being, despite her being so grateful for having her own space to live away from her ex-partner. Her struggle to live in this environment was particularly relevant given the freedom and space she had experienced during her own childhood in the Congo, and recognising this helped her to be more accepting of herself when she struggled with inner-city living. As a Muslim and someone who had grown up around beliefs in witchcraft, she valued the space to talk about the importance of her faith and this was a link to her parents and early childhood memories of them. We were able to explore aspects of her spirituality and childhood beliefs and practices that were both helpful and unhelpful for her currently. She felt that her faith became stronger during this time, which was a step to her linking to a local women's group in a mosque.

Fatima drew the tree diagram (Figure 5.2: Case study Tree Diagram) and she enjoyed naming goals, dreams and talents as well as labelling her resources and valued friends. This enabled her to more intentionally draw strength from these different positive aspects in her life. This prompted her to find an old friend and neighbour via Facebook who had been like a mother figure to Fatima when she and her partner had first come to the UK. She renewed this friendship and they began to talk regularly online. Fatima defined her overall life mission as being 'to grow and to learn in safety' and this was evident during the course of therapy.

The work was led by the issues that were brought to therapy each week, rather than using a more structured approach, and so it did not follow the weekly sessions of the Free to be Me course. However, this shows an example of how the key elements of HCBT can be integrated into therapy and used in an individualised way.

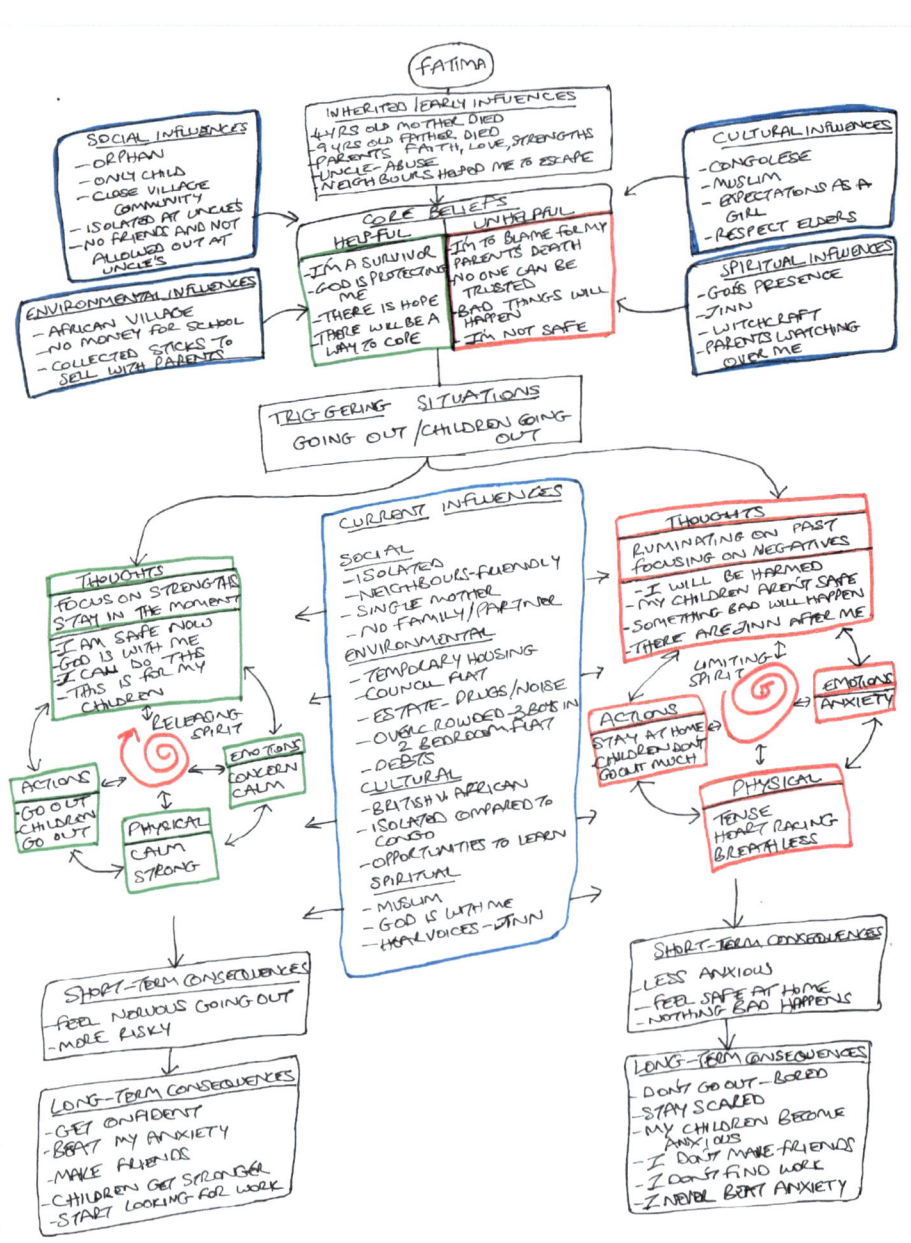

Figure 5.1: Case study formulation

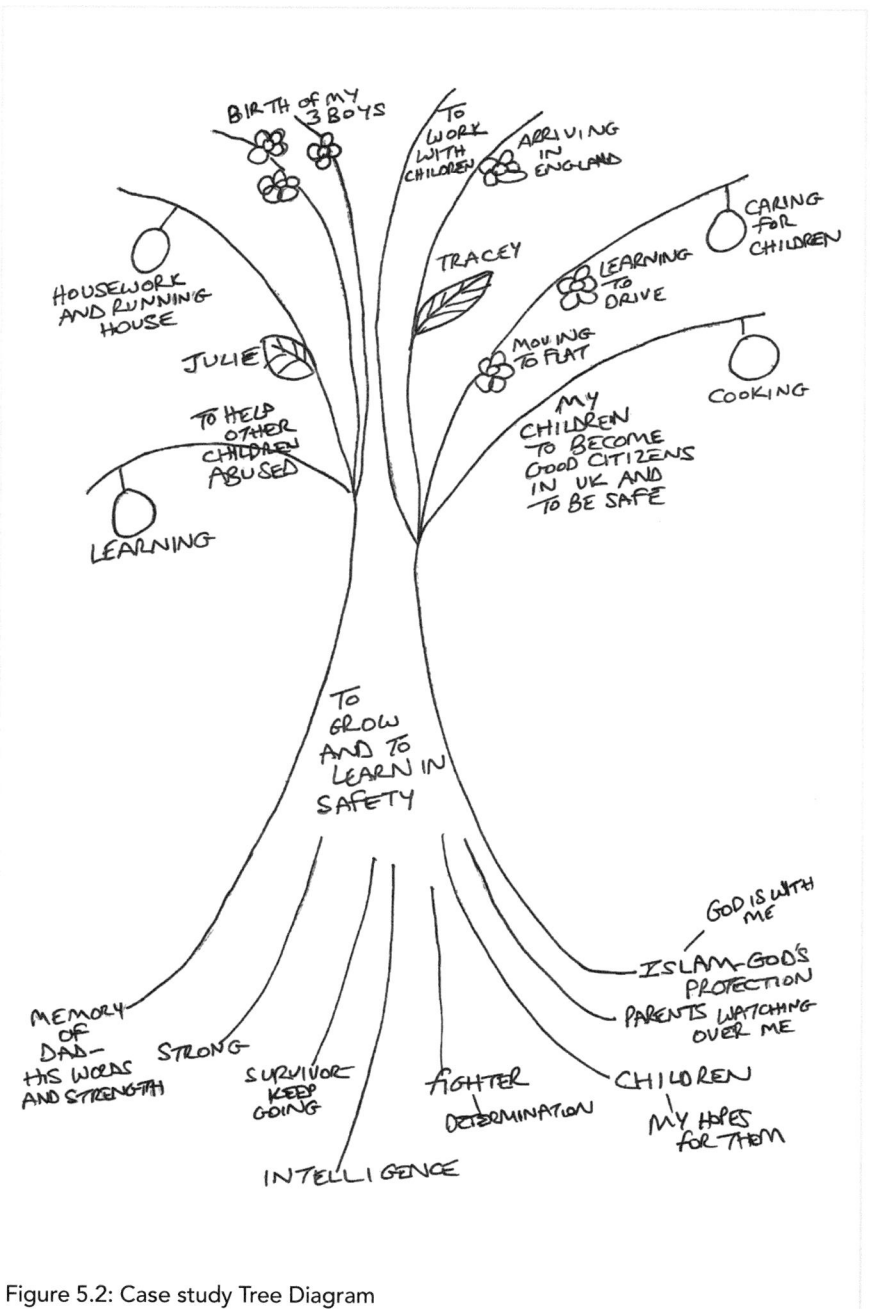

Figure 5.2: Case study Tree Diagram

Chapter 6: The process of HCBT

So, we have now covered the HCBT model and focused on the concept of the spirit before moving on to explore the developmental model of HCBT. This chapter now looks at how these ideas are used in practice, and in particular how they link to the Free to be Me course. These models are helpful to keep in mind when practicing HCBT but how the models are used is equally important to the models themselves. There is a danger in CBT that the models and formulations take precedence over how CBT is conducted, and though it is important to have these clearly in mind, we also need to ensure that the client feels heard and they engage with the process. If we use CBT in too much of a mechanical way without personalising the model, then it will not connect with the person sitting in front of us. The art of good CBT is to have such a clear understanding of the model in mind that we are able to weave it into the conversation so it is seen as personal and relevant to the client, using their own language and starting from their own understanding of their difficulties instead of starting from our own understanding. A good therapeutic relationship encourages the client to share honestly who they are. This will then help to create a better understanding for both therapist and client and help develop a holistic formulation of both their problems and their strengths that is truly co-created and personalised. This can then form the basis for the client to fully engage with the therapeutic process in a collaborative way.

The HCBT model and formulation is used explicitly within the Free to be Me course and over the weeks the participants work on different aspects of the HCBT formulation to gradually build up a personalised version of this. However, the HCBT developmental model is an underlying model which is referred to more indirectly depending on where people are at within this developmental journey. Having an understanding of the developmental model is similar to having an understanding of grammar when speaking English. It is really good to have that understanding of how grammar works in order to communicate clearly and to shape our words, but we don't need to explain the rules of grammar to someone in order to be understood. So, in using these models it is helpful to have them in mind in order for them to shape our communication and the direction of the work rather than the models dominating the process.

In order to look at the process of HCBT, we are going to focus on five key aspects of how to use HCBT. The first three aspects are more underlying aspects to the process, which are useful to keep in mind. These are: the holistic view of self; the key questions of life; and the goals of HCBT. The last two aspects are more about how we use HCBT in practice and consist of the group process and the role of the facilitators. The chapter concludes with a list of the overall HCBT principles to summarise the ethos of HCBT.

Holistic view of self

As we have seen already, each of us is a complex holistic whole with different physical, spiritual and psychological parts interacting with each other, as well as having a two-way relationship of influence with our wider context. Each of us is a wonderful, unique mix of complexity with strengths and weaknesses, with things we can endorse and strengthen within ourselves and things we want to change, and the whole is greater than the sum of the parts. It is important not to lose sight of this whole, but to help us to make sense of this bigger picture it can be useful to move our focus to these different aspects like moving a searchlight around to highlight different areas. HCBT is very much a balancing act of seeking to keep the whole person in mind whilst focusing on one part at a time. With each focus of the spotlight, it is then also about bringing it back to how that one part influences the whole and its impact on the wider picture. The Free to be Me course acts as a tour guide to explore each area in turn so that the participants gradually create a clearer map of their internal and external worlds. There are eight aspects of self which are helpful to keep in mind as we offer HCBT.

We have already explored most of these in previous chapters but this summary acts as a reminder of what has previously been said as well as serving to highlight a few other aspects of self. Within each section there will be reference to how they are explored within the Free to be Me course. Figure 6.1: The HCBT model was introduced in chapter 2 but it can act as a useful reminder as we explore these aspects of the holistic view of self.

A. The physical self

This is the outer circle of the HCBT model (see Figure 6.1: The HCBT model) and relates to our physical bodies, and in particular to the physical sensations we experience in relation to our thoughts and emotions. The physical self also relates to the actions that then come from our thoughts, emotions and physical responses and together they form helpful or unhelpful cycles. Behaviours that are a healthy response are in line with, and help to free, our spirit, and the more we act this way the more we are strengthening healthier versions of our self. In a similar way, when we act in unhelpful ways this limits our spirit and can lead to unhealthier versions of self being developed and strengthened.

A key exercise which is used to explore these ideas of freeing and limiting the spirit is the 'Review of the Day' exercise based on the Examen. This was mentioned in Chapter 3 and is introduced in Session 2 of the Free to be Me course. The exercise suggests reflecting on the day and noticing what energises us and what drains us. This simple exercise can be very useful in helping us to be more aware of the activities we do that are connecting us with our spirit and giving us a sense of flow and energy and which activities do the opposite. Helping people notice this change in energy levels within their body can be a key way of discerning when they are connecting with their spirit and living from the centre. At the end of each session on the course there is time given to complete a journal sheet and within this is a question about what resonated for them from the session. This idea of reflective journaling is another way to encourage people to look out for physical reactions to things from the course and to reflect on their significance.

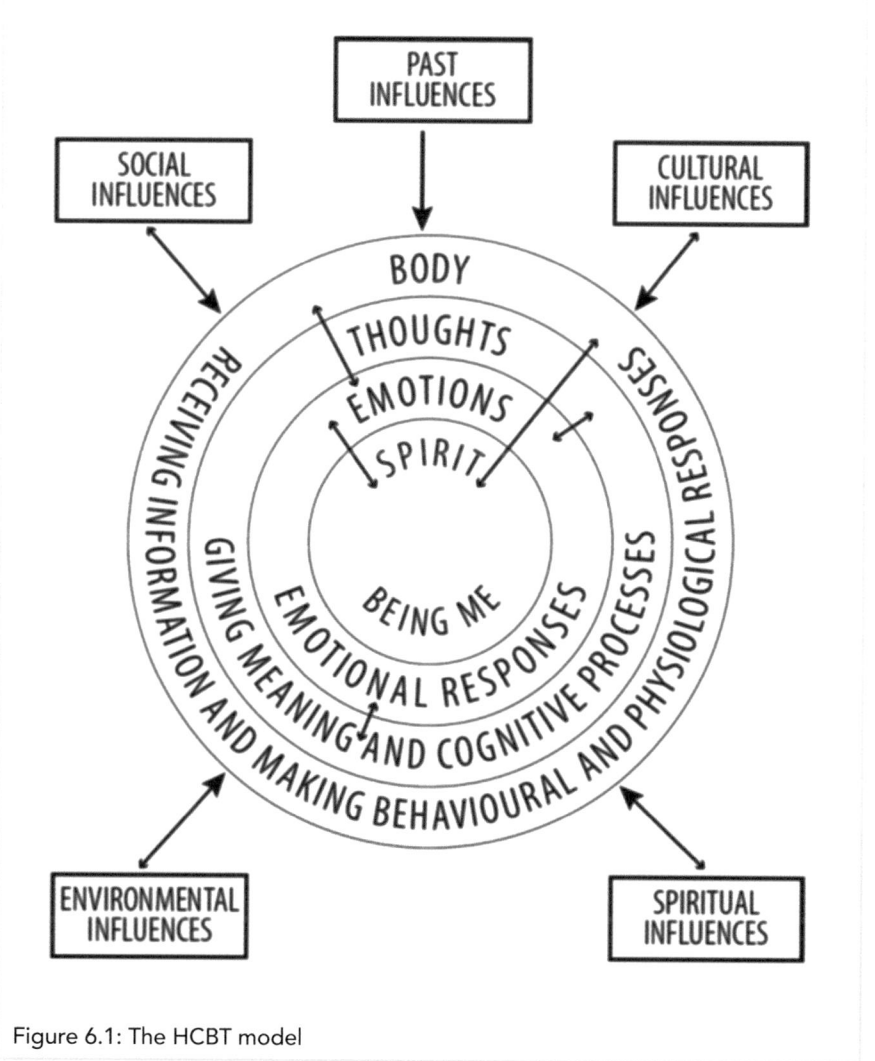

Figure 6.1: The HCBT model

Being aware of our physicality is an important part of HCBT and as a holistic approach it emphasises the body-mind-spirit link. The influence that our physical well-being exerts on our psychological and spiritual well-being is mentioned a number of times in the course but particularly in Session 10, which is the session which focuses on the body. In this session we encourage people to reflect on their bodies and to value them as more than just containers of who we are. The session encourages us to appreciate the amazing biology that keeps us alive and functioning and to develop a greater sense of appreciation for our bodies – including our imperfections. We review basic self-care such as good sleep hygiene, healthy eating and the importance of exercise as well as discussing the use of medication and herbal remedies.

In being aware of our physicality, it also reminds us of our connection with the natural world around us. Our physical bodies are made up of the same physical elements that make up all the various species in the natural world. Session 13 introduces the idea of ecotherapy and encourages us to reflect on this connection, recognising we are one part of a complex ecosystem. This session encourages people to connect with nature more and, for a few participants who have grown up in cities, it can be the first time they have experienced walking through woods, seeing only trees and vegetation and nothing manmade.

As with many aspects addressed on the course, we do not have time to cover everything in detail but we highlight possible avenues that people may wish to explore further if they sense they are appropriate for them. One example of this is in the session on the body in which we introduce the idea of 'Focusing'. This is a psychotherapy approach developed by Gendlin (1978). He introduced the concept of the 'felt sense' as a bodily awareness of something that is out of one's conscious awareness and so is difficult to put into words. Focusing suggests that listening to the body and identifying these sensations may lead us to identify issues or emotions that need voicing and so help us to understand ourselves better.

Movement is another way to connect with our physical self and this can also help participants to engage more fully with the topic being discussed. In each session the group is encouraged to move at some point even if it is just to get into small groups or to move to another part of the room to do a different activity. This is why, if possible, it is good to run the course in a space large enough to facilitate this. Moving to another space or the act of walking may potentially give clients time to reflect and process the topic a bit more than if they stayed in the same place. Movement is used to reflect on the HCBT model at the beginning of Session 3 and even standing up to put a Post-it on the wall can help us to connect with something differently in the process of moving. The session on the environment, Session 13, involves more extensive movement with a walk in nature. Walking has been suggested as a way of processing memories (Danylchuk, 2015), which is potentially one of the added benefits of ecotherapy as it usually involves walking as opposed to sitting in a therapy room. NLP (Neuro-Linguistic Programming) is another psychological approach that, among other techniques, uses movement to encourage a different level of processing. There are a few exercises on the course that have been adapted from NLP such as the timeline in Session 11.

B. The psychological self

The next two circles in the HCBT model (moving towards the centre) are the thoughts and emotions that are part of the psychological self. As we explored in the previous section, these interact with our physical sensations and actions to develop helpful and unhelpful cycles within the HCBT formulation. However, the psychological self is a lot broader than just our thoughts and emotions and covers various psychological aspects such as memory, personality and our focus of attention. The Free to be Me course is a personal development course which very much focuses on the psychological development of a person, and so the focus on our psychological self is evident in every session.

The course incorporates a lot of standard CBT to help participants to explore the psychological self. In Session 3 we introduce the CBT thinking errors that are unhelpful ways of thinking (such as catastrophising and all-or-nothing thinking). In later sessions we use thought records, behavioural experiments, graded exposure and other CBT techniques to help people to make positive changes. However, each of these CBT ideas are adapted to incorporate the concept of the spirit and how this can be limited and strengthened by our psychological responses and how in turn the spirit can act as a catalyst for change.

C. The spiritual self

As we have already explored, the concept of the spirit is at the heart of the HCBT model and this is explored primarily in Session 4 in the Free to be Me course. Participants are encouraged to reflect on this concept and to find a personal way of identifying with it which is in line with their own spiritual and philosophical beliefs. The course provides a safe space for participants to be curious and reflective about their own spiritual journey and to reflect on the spiritual influences around them (which is included in Session 14). This provides an opportunity to reflect on their own spiritual understandings such as their image of God, and their own spiritual beliefs in relation to their families and cultures and how their spiritual understandings might have changed over time.

Because the course includes matters of a spiritual nature, it can attract people who recognise a spiritual side to life, and so participants often come from a range of faith and spiritual backgrounds. This is one of the aspects that can be particularly valuable in running the course because there can be a rich discussion with people sharing about their spiritual lives and how this interacts with their mental and physical well-being. As we noted at the beginning of this book, a focus on the spiritual is often absent in mental health services apart from perhaps being directed to a chaplain, but even then, conversations with a chaplain are not usually integrated into their overall care. However, there has been some progress made in this area in which chaplains have been recognised as healthcare professionals and in some trusts are included more in the care of clients. Participants on the course who belong to faith groups often report finding it difficult to talk about their faith within mental health settings and then find it hard to disclose about mental health issues within their faith group so they are caught up in a 'double taboo' situation. The course therefore allows a space to talk about the impact of their mental health on their faith, such as finding the social aspect of meeting to worship difficult to manage when depressed, or the pressure they feel that they should be able to cope better because they have their faith. It also allows people an opportunity to recognise how their faith can be a strength and a resource and to reflect on what aspects of their faith are particularly important to maintain during a mental illness as a positive resource and what needs to be put on hold during this time. For example, attending a quieter, shorter church service that needs less energy during times of depression or attending the service but not staying for refreshments afterwards.

Recognising that we have a spiritual aspect to our lives encourages the exploration of what energises our spirit and provides a way of exploring spiritual aspects of life such as having a sense of meaning and purpose in life and recognising that we are connected with something bigger than ourselves. By acknowledging that we are spiritual as well as physical and psychological beings, this provides a way of exploring the key questions in life in terms of identity, purpose and direction (which we will look at more thoroughly in the next section of this chapter). This focus tends to lead to a greater understanding and valuing of ourselves as unique and valuable human beings. This can be a key turning point for people, particularly if they have grown up being told that they are inherently bad or worthless. This focus can lead to more self-compassion and forgiveness towards themselves which in turn makes people more forgiving and compassionate to others.

The course gives opportunity for personal reflection and encourages people to develop reflective practices such as journaling, the Examen and mindfulness. This is used in order to listen more to their spirit and to develop ways to connect more with their spiritual self. The value of meditation is recognised within HCBT and the word 'meditation' actually comes from the Latin 'stare in medio', which means to stay in the centre. Meditation can offer a way of learning to live from this centre. There is also a recognition on the course of post-traumatic growth and how difficulties can shape us and help us to grow. This is seen particularly in Session 11 in which we explore the past and how there is the potential to find meaning in all situations.

The image of the tree is used throughout the course to help to define aspects of our spirit and to think about the resources that ground us and where we draw our strength from; the hopes and dreams we have that stretch us and help us to grow; the moments of joy that make us feel it is good to be alive; our life's purpose; the significant people and communities that enable us to develop and our talents and strengths. By recognising these different aspects, it can help us to connect more with them and move to being more authentic and having a more purposeful life.

D. The social self

HCBT is ideally carried out in a group but even if it is done as individual therapy, it is still relational. If it is possible, Free to be Me sessions begin with a meal or at least some short time for refreshments so that there is an opportunity for informal socialising as well as more structured group discussions. The value of group therapy is explored later in this chapter but at this point it is important to note that the group itself and the peer support it offers is very much part of the effectiveness of the Free to be Me course, as with any group programme.

The group acts as a microcosm of the wider network of relationships that we are part of outside the course and is a reminder that it is these relationships that influence, strengthen and challenge us. In particular, the first community we were part of was our family. For some participants this was not a safe or nurturing environment but was somewhere they were discouraged to develop their potential or voice their views. So, a therapy group can be seen to be a healthy version of family in which people can begin to find their voice and share their stories in a safe space. As Desmond Tutu has been quoted as saying:

> '…you can't be human in isolation; you are human only in relationships…. We need other human beings in order to be human. I am because other people are. A person is entitled to a stable community life, and the first of these communities is the family.' (Tutu, online)

Within the course, participants are encouraged to share their reflections and questions about each topic through discussions in pairs, small groups or in the group as a whole. Over time the group usually becomes close as they share their vulnerabilities and struggles, and they laugh together and encourage each other on their shared journey. Strong relationships often form and these sometimes go on beyond the time of the course. The facilitators play an important role here in modelling healthy relationships and in creating a safe environment. For some people this may be the first time they have felt safe enough to share certain aspects of themselves or tell parts of their stories.

A particular aspect of the course which helps in developing the social self is the 'Threes' that happens about halfway through the course. People are divided into groups of threes and then, from Session 7 onwards, they have about a quarter of an hour each session to meet in their Threes for peer support. This helps to form an even closer peer support network with the opportunity to share with a smaller number of people at a deeper level, without the facilitators' involvement.

The social context is part of the HCBT formulation and so this is an ongoing theme throughout the course recognising that most difficulties in our lives, as well as many solutions, involve other people. Within the course we explore what healthy relationships look like and briefly explore assertiveness skills and teach a stepped process of forgiveness. Session 12 is the session in which we particularly focus on the social self and part of this session involves people mapping out their social networks and reflecting on their current relationships.

At the end of the course we are aware that saying goodbye to the group can be particularly hard for some participants, and so the majority of Session 16 allows for a reflection of the shared journey and marking its end. In this final session we also signpost people to other networks and ongoing community support for those who would find linking to other networks a helpful way to manage the group coming to an end.

E. The contextual self

Related to the social self is the idea that we do not exist in a vacuum but in a context of social networks, different physical environments, various cultures and, for some participants, their spiritual beliefs. These different influences are explored throughout the course both in terms of how they influence us but also to consider ways in which we can have an influence on them.

For example, in Session 13 we focus on the physical environment and in particular we explore ecotherapy and the value of connecting with nature. As part of this session, we think about the places in which we live and consider the impact on our well-being from factors such as overcrowding, poorly maintained housing, noisy neighbours or drab surroundings. Often people have lived in situations that they have not considered changing or have felt powerless to address and these can be chronic situations which have gradually been chipping away at their sense of well-being. These discussions can sometimes raise more socio-political discussions about unemployment, unstable housing and the sense of powerlessness against the system. The group can often be a catalyst for someone to make some changes in their environment even if it is just starting to grow tomatoes on their balcony or redecorating a bedroom.

The course looks at the influences from family, culture and faith traditions, particularly in Session 14, such as drawing a family tree and reflecting on how our beliefs and worldviews have been shaped by our wider context. The influence of the media – and especially social media – often comes up in these conversations. As with many issues on the course, it is becoming aware of these influences that helps people make informed choices. Some people begin to recognise influences for the first time and start to consider whether they find these influences helpful or not in terms of their personal development and well-being and whether any change is possible.

F. The developing self

The course follows a progression towards completing a full HCBT formulation and takes the group on a journey round different aspects of themselves. In this process there is a sense of development which mirrors the life journey that people are on. Woven into the sessions is an ongoing theme of personal development and growth and working towards goals and a sense of moving on in life. Session 5 in particular focuses on our goals, but also importantly focuses on our dreams and encourages people to explore these dreams seriously. If that feels too beyond their reach, then they can at least identify more attainable goals in line with these bigger dreams.

Session 11 focuses on our past, and participants draw a life map of their lives to reflect on their past and their life's journey. This can be a difficult process for those with traumatic pasts but they are given freedom to record what they wish to and how they represent it. So, for example, those with particularly difficult pasts may wish to represent difficult life experiences with a large dark cloud and leave it at that. This exercise enables people to review their life as a whole and to consider how they have developed and been shaped by their past. It may highlight patterns that keep repeating which need exploring further or past hurts that need some attention. Other exercises are used on the course to help people to reflect on their development such as the window exercise in which they draw images to represent their past, present, feared future and hoped for future in four sections in Session 7 and the timeline exercise in Session 11. There is also a similar exercise about how our spiritual beliefs and practices might have changed over time from our childhood to the present day. These exercises can sometimes be difficult because people reflect on their pasts which can contain painful memories but can sometimes also bring a sense of gratitude for the way things have happened. They can also encourage people to have a greater sense of agency to work towards a certain planned future rather than be passively shaped by the effects of past events.

The concept of time is explored briefly on the course in terms of where we tend to focus our attention; are we always forward-thinking either by being too driven by goals or future worries or are we dwelling too much on the past instead of valuing the present? The concept of mindfulness is introduced in Session 7 to encourage people to be more aware of the present moment.

The developmental model of HCBT is integrated within the course so that participants are working towards more helpful cycles and more helpful ways of being. This in turn is developing the healthier versions of self for each participant so they feel more integrated internally and externally. This process helps participants to be more aware of the influences around them as well as feeling more accepting of themselves in order to develop into more authentic, whole individuals. How far a person goes on this journey will vary from person to person and it will depend on their starting point at the beginning of the course. For some it may be developing into a more independent, assertive person who is starting new activities and new relationships. For another, meanwhile, it may be that they are already feeling that they have achieved these things in life and they are at the stage of letting go of responsibilities and activities and developing a slower pace and perhaps developing more spiritual practices.

G. The balanced self

The balanced self follows on from the developing self as something we are working towards. This is the focus of Session 15 and we use the ancient Celtic image of a trefoil to represent a balanced life: being, doing and learning. This also represents the balance between giving time to ourselves and giving time to others. Some participants have never felt they could have 'me-time' and so gaining a better balance of valuing themselves enough to rest and do things they enjoy can, for some, be quite revolutionary. Time management is part of this too and is briefly addressed in this session.

As we think about developing a better understanding of ourselves, this is also about getting a more balanced view of ourselves. Because the course is based on a holistic model, focusing on different aspects of ourselves helps to develop a more rounded, balanced view of who we are. For example, for those who tend to focus more on what they feel, there is the challenge to identify what they also think and for those who are more focused in their heads, they are encouraged to connect more with their emotions and physical sensations. Those who are more planners, may experiment with being more spontaneous and those who thought they were academic rather than creative may discover a more creative side. This is highlighted in session 12 when we explore personality types. This more balanced view of ourselves can in turn lead to a more balanced view of the world around us and the people in our lives – seeing both the helpful and unhelpful, the positives and the negatives.

H. The creative self

HCBT encourages the use of creativity as a complementary way of personal expression and reflection alongside the group discussions and teaching. CBT is predominantly a 'left brain', verbally-focused therapy that divides things into boxes, and so the use of creative exercises in HCBT encourages a more balanced approach. The work of Iain McGilchrist (2009) on the different roles of left and right hemispheres, mentioned in Chapter 2, highlights how biased our society has become towards the mechanical, pigeon-holing role of the left hemisphere which is good at mapping and analysing specifics. However, in doing this, the left hemisphere can struggle to see the bigger picture or make connections as the right hemisphere does, which is good at being able to make inferences, find meaning and accept complexity and mystery. There has therefore been a conscious awareness to encourage some right hemisphere activity within the Free to be Me course through creativity, reflection and the use of images, music and film clips. These creative exercises may be particularly appreciated by participants who find imagery easier to use than words and who would describe themselves as creative. People learn in different ways and some people are more left brain dominant and value lists of points on organised PowerPoint slides and to have group discussions, whereas others learn better through creative activities, movement and images. As we seek to be holistic, it is good to remember that we have both a left and right hemisphere in our brain and we need to engage our whole brains in our learning and development.

Symbolism and ritual are useful ways to connect with concepts and ideas at a different level. Symbols such as the tree can be helpful when we are trying to define something so enigmatic as the concept of the spirit. There are also aspects of ritual on the course such as developing the community tree alongside the individual trees. Sticking Post-its on a communal tree picture may not feel very ritualistic but there is a sense of familiarity as this becomes a group tradition which can act as a familiar ritual over the weeks of the course.

Usually within the group there are a few people who feel nervous about doing creative activities and worry about what their drawings will look like. However, we are all creative beings and with some encouragement people are able to tap into this perhaps more dormant side of themselves. If people are feeling hesitant about doing something creative for the first time in the group, we sometimes have a discussion about ways in which we are all creative but maybe don't recognise it – the person who likes to cook or garden, the person who finds creative ways of solving an issue at work or a parent who can keep a child occupied through various fun activities on a rainy day. People are encouraged to try some form of creativity but they will not be expected to share their results with the group. This helps to reduce any anxiety about using art materials, though in practice people often end up sharing their creations which they often find very affirming.

Images stay with people often longer than words and so imagery and metaphors are used quite often such as visual images to represent the spirit, the lantern image to represent the HCBT model and the developing tree image that they add to over the sessions. Creative activities give people the opportunity to reflect about an issue on their own as well as creating a visual reminder of these reflections, such as the life map, the window and the hand image they draw for healthy living goals. There is a lot of research to support the therapeutic value of expressive writing (Pennebaker & Smyth, 2016) and this is used on the course. Journal writing is used to reflect on each session and flow writing is introduced in Session 15. This is used to reflect on the course as a whole but is also offered as a tool to process any life events or issues.

Within the sessions, there are suggestions of film and TV extracts to play in order to help to illustrate points. These often act as good conversation starters. Again, these images stick in people's minds far better than any PowerPoint slide and can help to reinforce the focus for that week, as well as adding some humour and lightness to the session.

Playfulness and fun is encouraged, particularly when we are outside for the ecotherapy aspect of the course. People reconnect with childhood memories of fun activities when they are outside and this has led to groups enjoying playing on a swing and making a pile of Autumn leaves to jump in!

Another aspect of creativity is the Free to be Me playlist of songs. These tend to be from the last few decades of popular music which relate to the themes of the course, such as True Colours, Three Little Birds and Something Inside so Strong. This is played as people come in, over the meal and in breaks. People have fed back about the significance of those songs and how they have been reminded about the course in hearing the songs after the course has ended.

The key questions of life

As we run the Free to be Me course it is useful to keep in mind the underlying questions that may have brought the participants there. At the pre-course assessments, clients are asked what they want to be different or what they want from the course and they often say they want to be happy. When asked more about what life would look like for them if they were happy or if things were different, they usually give what seem to be the standard expected answers of wanting to work, have their own place or be in a relationship. These are genuine desires that are often very important to people; goals that they see as 'being normal'. But sometimes when they are asked whether they have any dreams for their lives, what they really want from life, what their ambitions were as a child, and if there were no obstacles in the way, what would they love to do, this is when clients are more likely to become animated and, with a spark in their eye and an excitement in their voice, they talk about something which is more specific to them; something that makes them feel alive and what would make life worth living again.

So, clients often come to therapy with the questions of how they can be happier or what can they do to reduce their anxiety, whereas when we broaden the focus and ask different questions they begin to connect with their deeper self. This is when the issue of reducing symptoms seems to become less important compared to what really matters to this person. These sorts of questions begin to connect with what is life-giving for that particular person and part of the process of HCBT is to help people to connect with any sparks of life that can be fanned into a flame in order to raise motivation. What do they really long for or really want in their heart? What really keeps them going when all hope is gone? And how can we build on that and help them to connect with that more? As we discussed in Chapter 1, in CBT and in most NHS therapeutic work, the focus is on reducing symptoms; helping people to feel less depressed or anxious – but then what? They may get less depressed or anxious but then there is the danger of being left with underlying questions of who they are and what they will then do with their life.

Some people may never feel that they have been in touch with their own desires or needs, particularly if they have experienced multiple traumas, loss and abusive relationships, and so they have never had the chance to develop healthy identities. Many clients who have been involved in mental health services long-term are in danger of seeing their identity wrapped up with services – they see themselves as patients before seeing themselves as individuals and their symptoms can become a key part of their identity. This lack of a sense of self is particularly seen with those diagnosed with Emotionally Unstable Personality Disorder in which there is a sense of never really knowing who they are and feeling like there is no constant, stable sense of identity.

For therapy to be holistic it needs to face the two key questions that can sometimes underlie people's psychological difficulties; firstly, who am I? And related to this are the questions, 'Am I of worth? And where do I fit?' These are the questions of identity, value and belonging. Secondly, there is the question of meaning and direction – what is the point of my life? Why am I here? And where am I going?

Erikson (1959) described eight stages of psychosocial development that an individual goes through as they mature, and at each stage he identified a key existential question. According to Erikson, it is during adolescence and our teenage years that we most ask the question 'Who am I?' and 'Who can I be?' However, this can be a question that continues through a lot of our adult lives and may particularly rise again during middle adult life when we may review how we have seen ourselves and who we are up to that time. According to Erikson, it is in middle adulthood that we ask, 'Can I make my life count?' and the questions of finding meaning and purpose in life are brought into focus. These stages reflect the developmental HCBT model of self which we explored in Chapter 4.

Who am I?

As far back as when Socrates stated, 'Know thyself,' and the Ancient Greeks were encouraged to 'become what you are', people have had a desire to know who they are and to feel that they are being true and authentic to that self-image. The question 'Who am I?' has many aspects and how we view ourselves is so important to our well-being, and should therefore be a key part of any therapy.

There is first the generic answer to the question 'Who am I?', and wondering about ourselves in terms of our generic psychological and spiritual makeup as people. There are different understandings about our internal makeup, and different therapeutic schools of thought reflect this. For example, psychodynamic therapy based on Freud's teachings sees our internal makeup based on various drives and impulses that are often in our unconscious. Jung's work focused more on the idea of a collective unconscious shared by the human race and surfacing in shared imagery and symbolism. Systemic thinking focuses on who we are in relation to others and that we are a combination of our internal worlds and the relationships we have with others. CBT is based on cognitive therapy which developed alongside the development of computers and equated our internal workings to computers; filing away stored memories like documents, some of which may be stored at different levels of awareness. As we have already discussed, cognitive behavioural understandings of identity focus on internal cognitions and how they interact with behaviours, emotions and our physiology.

We then have a specific question of who we are in terms of our personal sense of self and individual identity. This is about knowing what we tend to like and dislike, what we value and what is important to us – creating our external self which we discussed in Chapter 4. Our specific identity includes how we tend to act in certain situations and the roles we tend to have. There can be a process of questioning what is authentic to us and finding what naturally resonates with us, as we discussed in the last chapter. Some people find personality tests, such as the Myers Briggs Type Indicator and the Enneagram, helpful in identifying the sort of person they are and knowing their related strengths and weaknesses. Our sense of self is usually shaped by our background and life experiences – some of us choosing to be shaped in line with them whereas some of us may react against them. Our culture, ethnicity, socio-economic background as well as our physicality and sexuality as well as our spiritual and philosophical beliefs all have a part to play in shaping who we are, as does our ancestral and genetic makeup. Various aspects of our identity may surface as we ask this key question of identity. Figure 6.2: Who am I? highlights just some of the possible avenues where this question could lead.

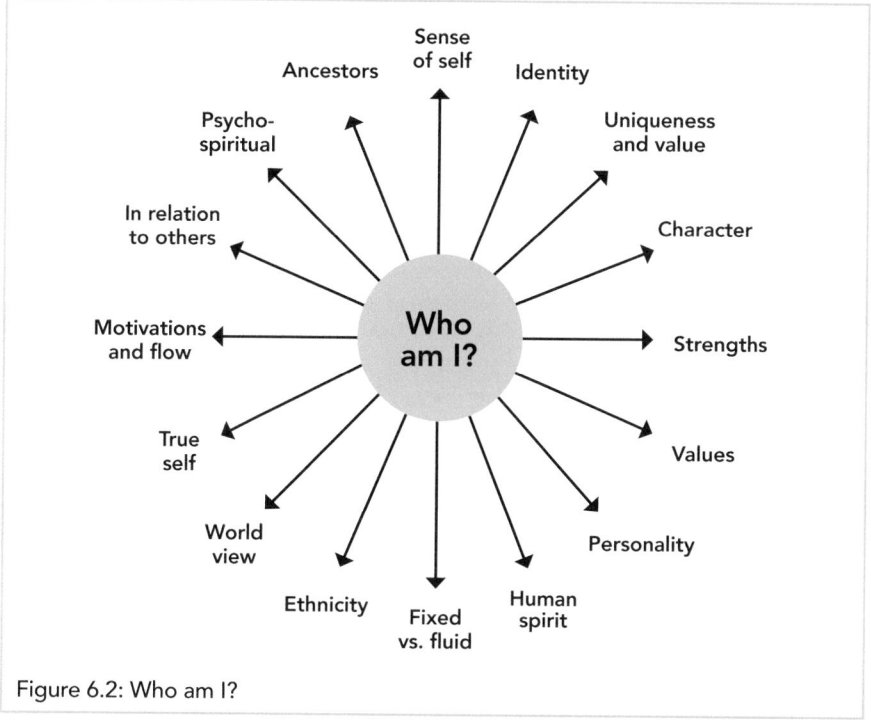

Figure 6.2: Who am I?

As we begin to understand ourselves, the next stage is accepting ourselves and ideally even liking ourselves. Many clients find it hard to engage with therapy because they do not believe they are worth changing and so this may involve a gradual process of trusting that what they hold within their identity is of value.

This question of 'Who I am' also connects with the question, 'Where do I belong?' It leads us to ask about belonging and the people and communities where we feel most at home. Understanding who I am helps to define who I feel drawn to and where I feel I fit in relation to significant relationships and to groups of other individuals where I feel a connection.

Where am I going?

Once we start defining ourselves with certain strengths, weaknesses, values and interests, then the next question arises: where am I going? This is about trying to make sense of the world – what does this thing called 'life' mean to me and why am I here? It leads people to wonder, 'If there is a person like me with this unique combination of attributes, what am I supposed to be using them for and how can I best use who I am in the world in which I live?' Finding a purpose in life and a sense that we can contribute in a meaningful way to a bigger picture or cause is good for our well-being. It is obviously also useful for those who benefit from what we give to others. If we are doing what we are naturally good at doing, then we will be in, what positive psychologists call, a state of flow and that feels good. As the philosopher, Nietzsche said:

'He who has a why to live can bear almost any how.'

This also ties in with the work of Victor Frankl who wrote a book (Frankl, 1959) based on his experience in a concentration camp. Frankl went on to develop logotherapy, which is based on the idea that life has meaning and we each need to find our own meaning in life, whether that is through a relationship, meaningful work, a purpose of some kind or, when all freedom seems removed, to have the freedom to choose our attitude and response within times of suffering. For those who have worked with people struggling with suicidal thoughts, it is difficult to challenge those self-destructive beliefs if people cannot connect with a reason to live and a sense of purpose. So helping clients to connect with meaning and purpose serves as a good antidote for those times of dark depression and when suicidal thoughts might surface.

The question of our life's purposes, again, has many facets, as shown in Figure 6.3: Where am I going? This sense of purpose relates to the goals in therapy which we will mention in the next section. If someone has a sense of their unique qualities and what they could use them for, then they are going to be motivated to work at reducing depression and anxiety and other barriers in order to do this. It is also important to remember that each of us will have multiple abilities and therefore various directions a person could take in life rather than just one particular path; so if one door is closed then there will still be other avenues to develop. By incorporating these ideas into therapy, clients can see a more fulfilling goal than just reducing symptoms because they are working towards being who they know they can be and doing what feels right for them.

Finding our individual purpose and direction can be difficult if this does not conform to other people's expectations; what the family expects or what social media advocates as a good life. As Shakespeare advised, 'to thine own self be true', and as Anthony de Mello says, the person who is able to live their own authentic life, independent of social pressures is:

'…a person who no longer marches to the drums of society, a person who dances to the tune of the music that springs up from within.' (de Mello, 2011)

A Radio 4 programme entitled 'The Wrong Job: Square pegs in Round Holes', suggested that up to 60% of people in the UK were in jobs they didn't really like or felt well suited to (BBC online, 2018). Therefore, there is the possibility that some people attending therapy for depression or anxiety may be experiencing these symptoms because they are not in careers they are well-suited to or not fulfilling a deeper purpose in their lives. Therefore, any amount of therapy is not going to help change this if it doesn't address this underlying issue. This could also apply to any number of life choices such as choice of partner, friends, leisure activities or home locations. Knowing who we are and what is important to us is therefore paramount in making any life choices and in developing our well-being.

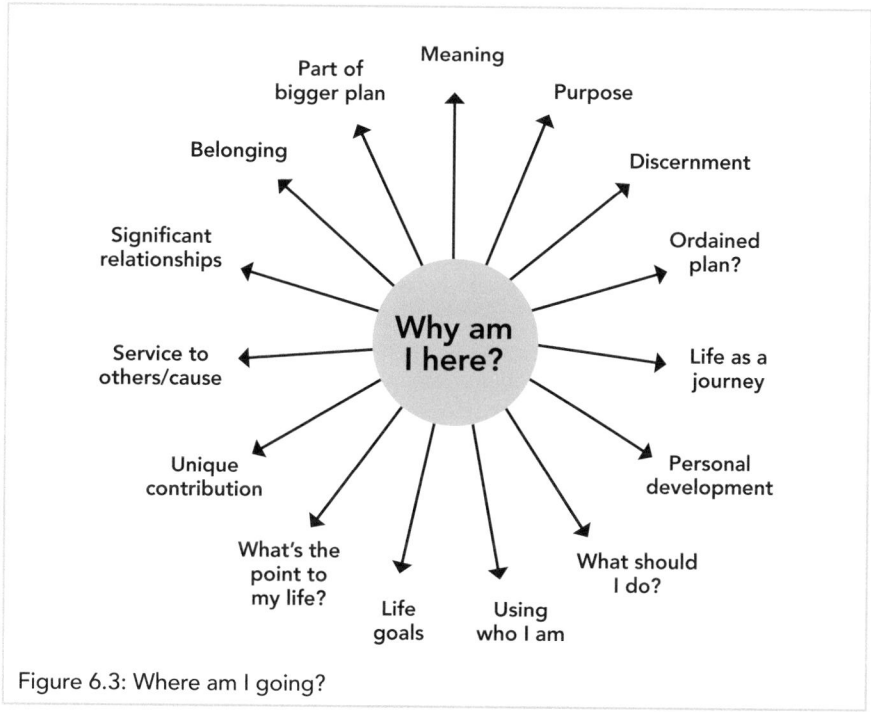

Figure 6.3: Where am I going?

In terms of purpose and meaning in life, what we do with our time is also going to have a significant impact on our well-being. If we are using our character strengths, if we are having periods of flow, if our work is in line with our values, then this is all going to increase our well-being. In particular, looking beyond ourselves and feeling connected to some form of larger purpose is going to help us to feel fulfilled. In Tom Rath's book *Life's Great Question; Discover How You Contribute To The World* he writes:

> 'A growing body of evidence suggests that the single greatest driver of both achievement and well-being is understanding how your daily efforts enhance the lives of others. Scientists have determined that we human beings are innately other-directed, which they refer to as being "prosocial." According to top researchers who reviewed hundreds of studies on the subject, the defining features of a meaningful life are "connecting and contributing to something beyond the self." (Rath, 2020)

A useful concept to think about our purpose is the hedgehog principle developed by Jim Collins (Collins, 2001) based on the idea that the hedgehog has just one way to survive – rolling into a ball – but that one strategy works well. In a similar way, Collins suggests that we can find a single strategy that works for us. He suggests that our ideal work is where three circles converge: what we love to do, what we are good at doing and what the world needs and is willing to pay us to do. (We explore this hedgehog principle in Session 15 of the Free to be Me course.)

HCBT seeks to give people space to explore these big questions in life using various methods to explore people's personalities, values and to reflect on who they are. As part of the HCBT process it is useful to be alert to these questions and to encourage discussion and reflection on them as they naturally arise.

Goals of HCBT

As with any therapeutic process, the goal of HCBT is about reducing symptoms such as depression and anxiety and improving well-being. However, as we have just said, these should not be our only focus. Within HCBT, the therapy also helps participants to find what motivates them and gives them a sense of purpose. So, as we have said before, a reduction of symptoms can be more of a by-product of learning to understand and accept ourselves and working towards goals that are in line with who we truly are. So, connecting more with our spirit would help us to focus away from our unhelpful thoughts and behaviours and to develop behaviours in line with our spirit and so feel more at peace with ourselves. Although reducing symptoms might be part of a person's motivation to attend, the HCBT process is more about developing the person than solving a problem and about developing well-being as a whole. A key goal in HCBT is therefore to help people to develop the art of listening to their spirit and discerning what feels right for them in terms of life choices, the roles they have and day-to-day decisions.

HCBT encourages people to explore childhood dreams and this can be useful in order to connect with their deepest dreams. This can lead to finding ways that they may fulfil the key aspects of this dream even when their actual dream is unattainable. For example, a person may have wanted to be a doctor but they now know that this is beyond them, academically. However, they may recognise that it is the aspect of care that was at the heart of this dream and so this can then lead them to find other ways to show care for others.

So HCBT aims to reduce symptoms, help people to understand themselves and rekindle past dreams, and helps people move towards wholeness. A useful concept when we are considering goals in a more holistic sense is the Hebrew word 'Shalom' in the Judeo-Christian tradition or the Arabic word 'Salaam', used in Islam to describe wholeness. Shalom or Salaam are interpreted as 'peace' in English but this does not do full justice to the breadth of meaning of these terms. It is actually a more active, dynamic word representing vibrant life and being part of a dynamic, living network of relationships in perfect harmony. The meaning of shalom represents everything in its right place and in balance, a person totally how they are meant to be, at peace with themselves and with those in their family and community. Shalom is not the absence of difficulties or unrest, but it is the sense that there is completeness, well-being and wholeness in body, mind and spirit, and also within relationships, within our physical environment and being at peace with ourselves and with the divine. The verb 'shalem' means 'to complete' and 'to make an end of', and implies that the process to shalom can be difficult and challenging in that total shalom needs to be reached for the whole and not just for an individual or a certain group within society. In that sense we may have 'peace' in isolation but not 'shalom'. Shalom implies that we are in healthy relationships with others and with our wider environment so we cannot have complete shalom if those around us and the natural world is not also experiencing shalom.

All areas of life are potentially reviewed during the course, even those that are functioning well, in order to develop goals of maintaining what is helpful as well as making changes to what is not helpful and to review life as a whole in terms of balance and well-being. HCBT therefore focuses more on what is working well compared to standard CBT which is more problem orientated and focusing on what needs to change. This leads to various goals that people may be working towards within the Free to be Me course – some may be learning to accept themselves more, some to be more mindful and less stressed, some may want to have the confidence to try finding work or start something they have been putting off for years. The HCBT model places greater emphasis on the effects of the physical environment, physical well-being, spirituality and relationships than perhaps standard CBT does and so goals may include changing some of these aspects. The goals are as varied as the participants who attend, but often they are related to feeling better about themselves, finding a purpose in life and learning to manage day-to-day challenges in more healthy, constructive ways.

It is important that the goals are authentic to each participant and that these goals are not imposed by others in the group or by others within their social network, and in particular not imposed by the facilitators. There may be times that people follow goals that the group and the facilitators may question, but it is important that people are supported towards their goals even though they may not align to what others feel are right for that person. This is because sometimes people need to go down certain routes and this is part of the process of learning what is and isn't who we truly are, and wrong turnings can be equally important in our journey as finding what is right for us. We also need to remember that we can be wrong and misjudge a person, and we do not always know what is right for a person. So it is important that we follow the ethos of the model and respect people's personal journeys without judgement or trying to influence a person's direction or goals, and allowing people to follow their own inner compass.

It may be helpful at this point to look at the World Health Organisation's definition of mental health:

> 'a state of well-being whereby individuals recognize their abilities, are able to cope with the normal stresses of life, work productively and fruitfully, and make a contribution to their communities.' (WHO, 2003)

This seems a very healthy goal to have, and, interestingly, it shows a recognition of well-being within a community context. It also highlights that mental well-being is not about an absence of symptoms, which ties in with the World Health Organisations broader definition of health in general as:

> 'a state of complete physical, mental and social well-being and not merely the absence of disease or infirmity.' (WHO, 2003)

This can be an important revelation for people who have been saying for years that 'when I get better then I'll do…' So another goal might be to help people to recognise what they can change and encourage them to work on those things, but also to help them identify what they can't change and for them to accept these things. People can therefore work towards life goals and lead fulfilling lives, even with physical or psychological difficulties, which has been a key message from the recovery movement within mental health services.

There are also indirect outcomes from the group that are not original goals but unplanned bonuses, such as ongoing friendships which are formed and unexpected results. One example of this was from the first course that was run in East London, which consisted of a diverse group from a range of ethnicities including white British, Asian, Oriental and African backgrounds, as well as people identifying as atheists, Christians, Muslims and Hindus. Feedback from one of the participants from a white working-class background illustrated how preconceived ideas can change in this process. He was someone who would not have normally mixed with people of other faiths and cultures despite living in a very diverse part of London and he said that through our discussions he had realised that, despite our varied backgrounds and beliefs, 'we're all quite similar, really'. That understanding of a shared humanity and a mutual respect for diversity was an important outcome for him personally and another step towards his own well-being in terms of changing perspectives of his wider social and cultural context.

Group process

As we have said, it makes sense to offer HCBT in a group format considering the importance of social context. The group dynamic is an added catalyst for change within therapy and there is a long history of research showing the value of group processes. In particular, Yalom & Leszcz (1985) identified 11 key therapeutic factors which help to explain why groups are so effective, such as instilling hope, a shared sense of universality, interpersonal learning and cultivating altruism. Morrison (2001) has more recently advocated for CBT to be provided in groups, particularly as a more efficient method. So although HCBT could be offered as an individual therapy, it would lack the therapeutic benefits of a group and so may limit its effectiveness.

The Free to be Me course is described as a personal development course in a group rather than being group therapy. Although there are elements of group therapy and space for people to talk, it is predominantly a psychoeducational course with PowerPoint presentations, handouts and activities. Unless a relational difficulty arises in the group which needs exploring directly within the group, relationship issues in the here and now are not part of the HCBT process as they would be in traditional group therapy.

Groups show a creative dynamic which is rarely seen to the same extent within individual therapy. This is a good example of when the whole is greater than the sum of the parts because a group of people can spark off each other to create new ideas and come to new conclusions. There are times when, as facilitators, we can feel the energy shift in the room as people focus on a particular topic of discussion through a comment made or the sharing of a story which feels alive and productive. This is when it is helpful to allow that discussion to unfold and see what emerges, because there is a cathartic process happening which is the group dynamic at play.

The group creates a community on a small scale through the shared meals, group sessions and the Threes for peer support. As a microcosm of life and of our wider society, groups can provide the ideal training ground for people to grow in confidence and to manage relationships better than if they were in individual therapy. People often come to groups feeling apprehensive and perhaps reluctant to trust others, but this is part of the process. People often feedback at the end of the course that it was being in the group that was the most rewarding part of the course; learning to be free to be themselves with others, trusting people and hearing that others have similar experiences.

Facilitators' role

Let's now explore the role of the facilitator within the HCBT approach. (We are using the term 'role' in a general sense here rather than in terms of external roles within the developmental HCBT model. However, you may find it helpful to reflect on your own roles and how this might help or hinder your role as a facilitator within the Free to be Me course.)

Shared Journey

An important premise for the facilitator's role is the recognition that group facilitators are, in a sense, also group participants. As practitioners of HCBT the person we are is as important, if not more important, than the techniques and theories we use. It is useful to remember that we are fellow travellers on a personal development journey towards wholeness and HCBT seeks to reduce the power difference between the 'us and them' within the therapeutic relationship. Where it is appropriate, it is helpful to share from our own journeys of self-discovery and recovery and share about our own struggles and times of growth. This needs to be done sensitively so that our stories prompt others to share rather than dominate the space, and it's important to be mindful of what will be helpful for those listening. In this way the facilitators can model and encourage openness and vulnerability.

As well as facilitators being participants, the reverse is true. The group participants have a role in the group facilitation in that they are shaping how the group is used by their input and feedback. The way in which HCBT is offered therefore encourages a sense of peer support and a recognition that there is not an 'us and them' as much as there is an 'us'.

As fellow travellers, HCBT puts greater emphasis on own growth as therapists and our own journeys than perhaps standard CBT would. As therapists, it is helpful if we can be in an ongoing process of our own self development, so that we can help others from a place of our own authenticity and genuine empathy, instead of helping others based on our own needs and motivations. In an ideal situation, there will be moments when the facilitator is speaking from their spirit, and then this is more likely to resonate with the spirit of those listening to encourage a deep connection and mutual openness. In those moments when people are connecting at that deep spirit level then change is more likely to occur, both within the facilitators and the participants, as Jung has said:

> 'The meeting of two personalities is like the contact of two chemical substances; if there is any reaction, both are transformed.' (Jung, 1933)

The transpersonal psychologist, John Rowan, talks about resonance between two people and likens it to two pianos both hitting the same note at the same time, and:

> 'that inner experience within the therapist during which he or she co-feels, co-enjoys, co-suffers and co-understands with the client.' (Rowan, 2005)

As HCBT facilitators, we are seeking to be whole people and modelling that holistic perspective. At the heart of HCBT is this idea of living more from the centre – connecting with who we truly are and speaking from the heart. Therefore, the ideal is for HCBT therapists to be facilitating the group in this way. This is therefore more than just reading a manual and following it step by step. It is also about listening deeply to what people are saying and listening to what seems to be coming from their spirit. So that when you hear something significant you can acknowledge and encourage it. This is why it is good for you, if you are facilitating the group, to have read the material and feel familiar with it. There are times when we really connect with someone even if we have only just met with them – there is a sense that we are on the same page, their experience resonates with ours and we feel free to share from our heart with them. This is what we want to aim to get to in the Free to be Me groups. What we say as facilitators is a small part of this process; it is how we say it that will often speak more to people. This also helps us to engage with the process more as facilitators and prevents it from becoming a dry exercise in which we simply read out of a manual. It will energise us as facilitators as well as energise the group. It is worth checking in with ourselves as facilitators every now and again about how we feel towards the group; are we showing compassion, do we believe that each of these people in the group are unique and valued and have something worth saying? The answer to these questions will affect how we speak to the group and also what we will hear.

Therapeutic listening and responding

Listening is at the heart of any therapeutic group and is an active process rather than a passive one. For those of you who have had any counselling or therapy training, you will be familiar with the basics of listening, and more importantly showing that we are listening through non-verbal cues and reflecting back what we have heard. If we consider the HCBT model of body, mind, emotions and spirit, we can think about listening at all these levels. The facilitator's aim is to listen to the person's emotions, their thoughts, to observe their body language and to listen out for things that seem to be coming from their spirit – what they connect with most deeply. As St Benedict wrote at the beginning of his monastic rule, we are 'to listen with the ear of the heart'. We are receiving information as listeners but we are also listening with our whole beings – what bodily and emotional reactions do I sense within myself as well as my thoughts and what connects with my spirit from what they are saying?

The following adapted quote from the Bloemfontein Samaritans, South Africa, is a good reminder of what true listening involves:

> You ARE NOT LISTENING to me when …
> You do not care about me
> You say you understand before you know me well enough

You have an answer to my problem before I've finished telling you what my problem is
You cut me off before I've finished speaking
You finish my sentences for me
You feel critical of my vocabulary, grammar or accent
You are dying to tell me something
You tell me about your experience, making mine seem unimportant

You ARE LISTENING to me when…
You come quietly into my private world and let me be me
You really try to understand me even if I'm not making much sense
You grasp my point even when it is against your own sincere convictions
You allow me the dignity of making my own decisions even though you think they might be wrong
You do not take my problem from me, but allow me to deal with it in my own way
You hold back your desire to give me good advice
You do not offer religious solace
You give me enough room to discover for myself what is really going on.

As well as listening, how we respond is key. It is helpful to be aware of the language we use as facilitators. Does it reflect the ethos of HCBT? Does it affirm the positives in people and encourage their individuality? It is important that our language is inclusive, being mindful of all the protected characteristics such as gender, race and sexuality, and does not discriminate in any way. It is also important to try and use language which fits with everyone in the group. For example, if people see the spirit in different ways or have different spiritual beliefs, then it is important to include these if we are talking about spirit. (This is why it is helpful in the assessments before the course to get some basic understanding of how a person may see their spirituality and what terms they identify with.)

We also want to be highlighting the strengths and the positives to balance the negatives. A useful therapy method is reframing, which can help to put a different twist to a situation. If used at an appropriate time, it can be helpful sometimes to 'reframe' a negative situation to see more positive aspects or to have a more balanced view.

Mutual learning

The group facilitators should try to encourage an environment of shared learning and openness rather than the idea that there is a 'correct answer' to things. This avoids a classroom-style learning in which facilitators are seen as teachers with knowledge. As the name 'facilitator' suggests, they are to facilitate the group to trust each other, to create a safe space and encourage mutual sharing and learning. This fits with the classic Socratic approach within CBT in which the style is to ask questions to help people to find their own answers rather than telling people what to think and do. Having said that, the course is quite didactic in its style but allows space for discussion and for personalising the material. As we look at various external influences that can shape who we are within the HCBT model, we need to be mindful as facilitators that we don't become another external influence that seeks to shape participants. Instead, we should allow them to make their own choices and to follow their own process of discernment, within a guided structure.

CBT encourages people to try out new things as a means of discovery, and it uses the idea of behavioural experiments to do this. As with any scientific experiments, there is the idea that there are no mistakes or failings – just learning from the last attempt and adjusting how it was done to try it again. This is used in HCBT and encourages curiosity and hopefully a willingness in the group to experiment with new things and to test things out without the fear of getting it wrong or making mistakes.

Celebrating diversity

Another of the facilitator's key roles is to celebrate individual difference, and when someone shares a strength that is personal to them it is helpful to reinforce and encourage this so that the person takes note of what that is. The recognition that diversity is part of the richness of life is highlighted throughout the course and the natural world's extensive diversity is a continual reminder of how drab life would be if everything was uniform. In a group of people there will be different perspectives and different life choices, and this is encouraged. We do not want to convey the message that there is a right way and a wrong way to live. This may seem to contradict the helpful and unhelpful cycles of HCBT, but it is each individual who determines what is helpful and unhelpful based on their own inner voice making that distinction rather than it being imposed on them by others.

Encouraging self-worth

HCBT seeks to focus on positives and strengths as much as, if not more than, unhelpful thoughts, behaviours and symptoms. This can involve helping people to visualise what healthy alternatives might look like. It is also about reinforcing positive behaviours by focusing more on them and exploring them instead of focusing on symptoms. Hopefully throughout the course people begin to develop a greater self-worth. To help with this the facilitators should be mindful of how they are responding to people in the group and whether they are showing unconditional acceptance to all group members. It is difficult for participants to develop self-acceptance if they don't feel that acceptance from the facilitators, and sometimes it is the role of the facilitator to see past the unhelpful aspects of a person to some of their core strengths. If we find that this is a challenge with a particular participant it is important to explore this with the other facilitators outside of the group. It sometimes needs talking through to understand what that particular participant might be triggering within us and to identify some of their core strengths and positive aspects.

One of the facilitator's roles is to look out for glimpses of the spirit within each person and help them to see these for themselves. It is important to highlight the moments when a participant recognises a strength, something they can do, something they like about themselves or when they feel connected to others or to something bigger than themselves. When these moments happen, the facilitators can help the person to recognise these things which resonate for them or they feel strongly about by reflecting them back and highlighting what they have said. As facilitators, be curious and ask more, rather than try to interpret these moments; encourage participants to ask themselves what has made them react in that way. It is useful to listen out for when someone is speaking about something for which they feel a real passion and which energises them. These are opportunities to ask more in order to help them to connect with how important this is for them and to reinforce their passion or ability. If someone talks about doing something which reflects a character strength or value that could also be highlighted and built on. By doing this we are using basic behavioural therapy to reinforce the positives and redirect the person's focus to their strengths and potentials in order for them to connect and develop these more fully.

Developing to our full potential

There is a process in HCBT of encouraging people to reach their potential, helping them to recognise their purpose and encouraging them to dream again.

So, the facilitators' role is also to keep in mind the person's long-term goals and encouraging them to reach their potential, and ultimately to find something to feel connected to beyond themselves, where this feels appropriate.

The developmental HCBT model can be helpful to keep in mind when running the Free to be Me course, particularly because it is not explicitly taught on the course but is only referred to indirectly. As facilitators, you may find it useful to recognise where people may be on this developmental journey; are they at the earlier stage of developing their 'glass lantern' – building a sense of self around their roles, their career and relationships? Or are they established in their sense of self in relation to these external aspects of life and are they at a phase of reflecting more deeply on their inner character and letting go of aspects of themselves that may not resonate with their spirit? You may also be aware of different roles that people move into, and you may notice how they use different roles at different times on the course. However, it is important that a person explores their own roles and identifies them for themselves instead of someone else pointing them out.

Despite this HCBT process being about understanding ourselves (whether as group participants or facilitators) we also need to recognise that, ultimately, we can never fully know ourselves and certainly not fully know others. We are each a complex, dynamic being and so as facilitators we cannot assume we know someone and so we need to keep an open, curious stance towards people in the group. As people we cannot be fully analysed and explained by medical science, psychological approaches, neurological studies or wisdom traditions. Even if we did know all about a person at any one moment, there is an ongoing development and dynamic state of flux occurring so that just when we feel we have grasped who this person is, they grow and develop beyond our full understanding including our own knowledge of ourselves. There is something about our dynamic whole and the essence of a person that remains elusive, and rightly so.

HCBT principles

The HCBT ethos has probably been evident as we've journeyed through the preceding chapters. However, to conclude the book, the following is a summary of the 20 key principles of HCBT:

1. Standard CBT along with third wave CBT offer many useful theories and techniques that are used in HCBT.
2. Along with a physical and psychological part to us, we also have a spiritual part that is represented by the concept of the human spirit.
3. Each person's spirit is the source of their potential and their deepest dreams, purposes and strengths that are specific to them. The more that a person discovers and lives in line with their spirit, the greater their sense of well-being and their spirit can act as a catalyst for change.
4. The HCBT process is about recognising unhelpful cycles that limit who we are and to create more helpful cycles that free who we are and to consciously choose to move into the helpful cycles.
5. The aim of HCBT is to live increasingly from the centre, from our spirit, and to respond to life instead of reacting to it.
6. We do not exist in a vacuum. As well as our past, we are influenced by our social, spiritual, environmental and cultural contexts and so it is important to explore these within the therapy.
7. We are social beings and relationships are key in shaping who we are and helping us to develop in becoming all that we could be, and so HCBT is best done within groups.
8. Each of us develops external versions of our self made up of different roles, and these help us to define our identity, build relationships and work towards goals.
9. Through various processes and therapeutic work we can discern what is from our spirit which helps to develop healthier versions of our self.
10. The more our external versions of self are developed in line with the spirit the more a person develops healthier versions of themselves. The

less these external versions of self are in line with our spirit the more we develop unhealthy versions of ourselves.

11. Each person is unique and valuable and is made up of a mixture of strengths, abilities, weaknesses and characteristics which no other person shares.

12. Because each person is unique, it is important to value difference and encourage group participants to share their views and respect each other's viewpoints, which in turn helps the group to gain a more holistic view of life.

13. Because we are all different, it is important to use a variety of learning methods within HCBT – engaging left and right hemispheres of the brain and using discussion, movement, creativity and reflection. Making space for creativity and laughter alongside discussion and quiet reflection helps to bring balance to the process.

14. If we live according to who we truly are, then this energises us whereas if we live according to unhealthy versions of our self, or in roles which don't fit with who we truly are, this can lead to burnout or a sense of emptiness.

15. HCBT recognises an interconnectedness internally, of body, mind, emotions and spirit, but also a connection within the wider network of life – in terms of relationships with other people, with the natural world we live in and with what some call God or a higher power and in HCBT is called Life's Source and Flow.

16. There is great value in connecting spirit to spirit with other people and having authentic conversations, and the HCBT group aims to be a safe space for this authenticity and speaking and listening from that deep place within us.

17. HCBT can be a way of exploring key questions in life of identity, purpose and belonging, and knowing that we each have value and a direction in life can improve our well-being.

18. The focus in HCBT is in developing the person more than just solving a problem and the strengths and potential of an individual need to be recognised as much as their weaknesses and their struggles.

19. HCBT aims to empower people and to encourage their own self-discovery.

20. HCBT recognises that, ultimately, we cannot fully understand ourselves or other people because we are each a unique, complex and dynamic being, and this adds to the richness of the journey.

Epilogue

How will HCBT develop in the future? I am hoping that, by sharing this holistic approach, it will be used by people in various settings from different professions and backgrounds. This will inevitably shape HCBT and develop it further. I also look forward to continuing to develop the ideas shared within this book within my own therapy practice. In CBT there are specific formulations for various diagnoses and so there is the potential for developing these formulations for presentations such as panic, OCD, psychosis and low self-esteem to include the spiritual, the context and helpful cycles. This will create more holistic formulations and therefore a more holistic approach to CBT.

Over the last few decades, there has been a growing awareness of the importance of mental health. This has been encouraged by various celebrities speaking out about their own battles in this area as well as numerous public health initiatives to raise awareness. This has particularly been the case during the national lockdowns throughout the Covid-19 pandemic and it is likely to be an ongoing focus as the UK, along with countries worldwide, begin to come out of the pandemic and reflect on the mental health impact of Covid-19.

Along with a growing awareness about the importance of mental well-being there seems to be a growing awareness within Western cultures that there is still a space for spirituality alongside the scientific developments of the last centuries. Increasingly, there is a recognition that we can integrate science and spirituality together and it does not have to be an either/or belief system. Again, the Covid-19 pandemic and its after-effects have raised existential questions about our values and what we want for the future of our nations and for the planet that we share. Within the field of psychology, there is ongoing interest in transpersonal and holistic approaches to therapy such as psychosynthesis, which is an integration of spirituality within a psychodynamic approach. By offering HCBT, I hope to offer a way to integrate spirituality within a CBT approach for those who wish to continue to work within a CBT model but who also wish to include a spiritual aspect to their therapy practice.

Within my own work, I have had the opportunity to teach ways in which spirituality can be explored and integrated within therapy, and this has led to the opportunity to teach HCBT in various settings such as with psychology trainees, GP chaplains and counsellors. I hope that HCBT might continue to be taught alongside standard CBT and third wave CBT approaches as another way to offer CBT. HCBT may be particularly appealing to those who wish to broaden the CBT approach and consider issues such as spirituality and ecotherapy as well as using creativity more within CBT.

My hope is that HCBT will continue to be offered within NHS mental health services and that it will become an option nationally in various mental health teams and counselling services. This is a time of significant change for the NHS as a result of the NHS Long Term Plan (2019). These proposals, along with developing many other areas of the NHS, seek to redesign mental health services to fit round the newly formed primary care networks of GP surgeries. This is in line with the Community Mental Health Framework for Adults and Older Adults (Sept 2019) in which it states:

> "This Framework sets out how the vision for a new place-based community mental health model can be realised, and how we can modernise community mental health services to shift to whole person, whole population health approaches."

HCBT offers a therapy that seeks to be more 'whole person, whole population' in its approach and so it fits well with the ethos of the Community Mental Health Framework. This framework encourages mental health services to be more preventative and to promote well-being as well as reduce ill health and also promotes a more strengths-based approach. The ethos of HCBT therefore sits well with this future direction of mental health services and supports the six main aims outlined in the framework, and in particular HCBT is aligned to the following aim, as quoted from the proposed framework:

> "[to] improve quality of life, including supporting individuals to contribute to and participate in their communities as fully as possible, connect with meaningful activities, and create or fulfil hopes and aspirations in line with their individual wishes."

The framework also promotes co-production and recognises the important role that service users can play in shaping and delivering services. With greater numbers of peer workers and those with lived experience joining the NHS work force, there is a growing recognition that there is less of a divide between 'patients' and 'providers', and that we are all on a continuum of mental well-being and on a journey towards wholeness. This development is gradually changing the culture of mental health provision and HCBT, and the Free to be Me course in particular reflects this recovery and enablement ethos. In particular, the Free to be Me course is a natural fit for a Recovery college setting, which provides courses run by Experts by Experience alongside healthcare professionals. It is hoped that the Free to be Me course will be offered in these settings as well as in other mental health settings.

As well as clinical settings, the Free to be Me course has been used in community settings as a personal development course, and it is hoped that HCBT offers a tool for CBT to be offered more widely in community settings within the new 'place-based community' model. The course offers a preventative, public health approach to mental health which would work well as a community psychology approach as well as being a more therapeutic intervention. It is therefore hoped that the course will facilitate CBT to be taught in various settings, which could include community centres, faith groups, hostels, retreat centres and addiction services. In particular, it would be interesting to see if the Free to be Me course could be used within schools, youth clubs and other settings for young adults and whether it can be adapted for different age groups.

Increasingly, mental health services are becoming more aware of being inclusive and culturally relevant. Services such as IAPT routinely analyse data in terms of who accesses their service and whether this is representative of the local population. Where ethnic minority (or more appropriately named, global majority) populations are underrepresented, some services are seeking to develop community psychology approaches to reach out to different communities. The Free to be Me course offers an ideal vehicle for a service such as IAPT to take CBT beyond the walls of the IAPT service to where people already meet within the local community. So instead of expecting everyone to come into services, IAPT staff could run a Free to be Me course in a community centre or in a place of worship and take CBT into the community. People are more likely to access a service within a more familiar setting and the course can be co-facilitated with members of the local community and adapted for the specific group attending.

The ethos of HCBT seeks to highlight the importance of interconnectivity and the importance of well-being for others as well as ourselves, and so may be suited to more collective, non-Western cultures as well as more individualistic Western cultures. In particular, it is hoped that it can be used in community settings within countries where access to mental health services is very limited. We are in the process of developing a Christian version and Muslim version of the Free to be Me course and it is hoped that these faith-based versions can be used within faith communities both in this country and in countries where mental health provision is harder to access. Within this country, the Christian version of the Free to be Me course has been piloted within a church setting and was attended by those from the church as well as those connected to the church through the foodbank and children's clubs. There are also plans to develop the Muslim version to be run within UK mosques and Islamic schools.

As well as changes within mental health services, there are changes within the business and organisational world. The work of Frederick Laloux, which is described in his book *Reinventing Organisations*, suggests how some organisations are beginning to change in their management styles and structures. He describes various case studies of successful businesses who have developed 'more soulful and purposeful ways to run business', where people are encouraged to shape their work round their individual skills and interests (Laloux, 2014). Laloux suggests that the future of organisations could be places where people can feel more authentic and feel that they can bring their 'whole self' to work and not hide behind professional personas. This approach encourages workers to reflect on their skills and interests and to consider, with their colleagues, where they would fit best within an organisation to not only develop the company but also develop their own potential. One of the contributory factors of burnout and of boredom is being in a job which does not fit a person's natural strengths and interests. Therefore, organisations which support staff to recognise and develop their personal strengths may help to reduce both burnout and boredom and increase their staff's commitment and enjoyment in work. The ethos of HCBT is in line with this development of bringing the whole self to work and could be used in the workplace to support such forward-thinking organisations. HCBT offers a tool for personal development and could be used within organisational staff support such as Employee Assistance Programmes and business coaching.

HCBT is about finding balance and well-being within ourselves, recognising and valuing the different inter-related parts that make up the whole. HCBT is about discovering our true self and developing this potential by letting go of unhelpful ways of being that hold us back and developing helpful ways of being. But this is not a journey of isolation but of interconnectivity. We are each one part of a larger whole and well-being comes from relationships; from our relationships with others, with nature and with Life's Source and Flow. This recognition of our interdependence and the importance of building these healthy relationships is needed not just for our own well-being but, in the face of Western individualism and global threats of climate change, for the well-being of the world.

I hope that HCBT is something that continues to be used and developed, and in line with HCBT ethos, I hope that those aspects of HCBT which are not helpful will fall away and those aspects that are helpful will continue to grow and be developed. If you use HCBT as a model of therapy or if you run the Free to be Me course, then please send any feedback, queries and stories of how you have experienced HCBT either as a participant or provider and I welcome your comments via the website: www.hcbt.co.uk

Dr Hilary Garraway, 2021

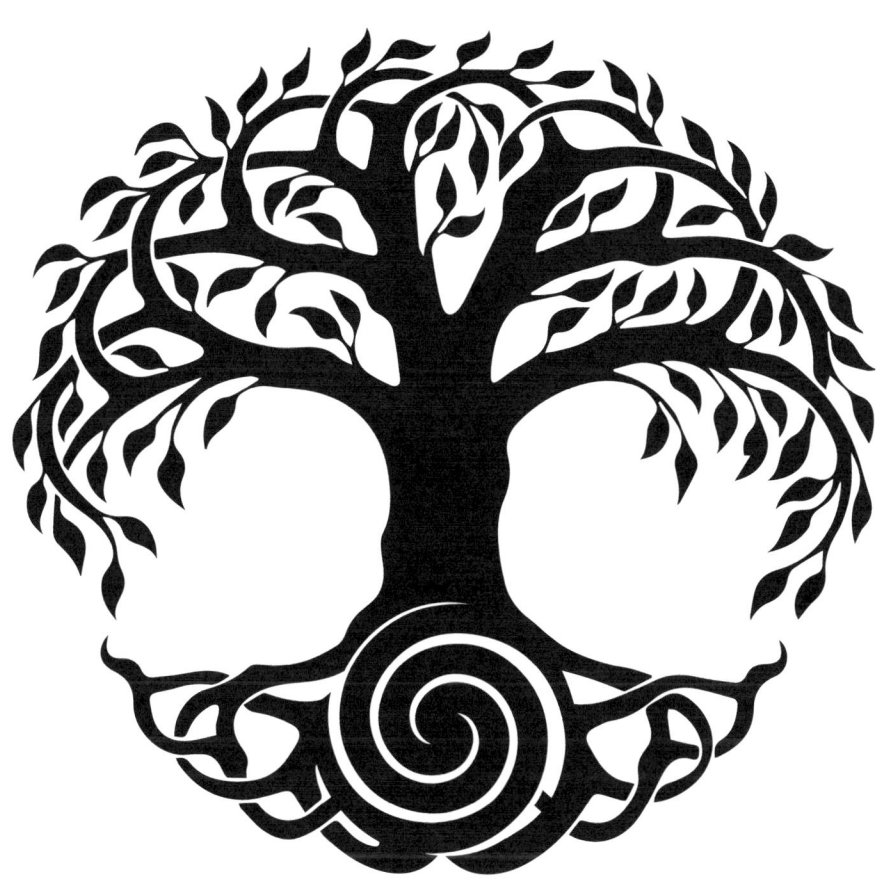

References

Assagioli, R (1965) Psychosynthesis: A manual of principles and techniques. Hobbs, Dorman & Co., Inc.

Avants, S, and Margolin, A (2004). Development of Spiritual Self-Schema Therapy for the treatment of addictive and HIV risk behavior: A convergence of cognitive and Buddhist psychology. Journal of Psychotherapy Integration, 14(3), 253-289.

Azhar, M & Varma, S (2000) Mental illness and its treatment in Malaysia. In I. Al-Issa (Ed.), Al-Junūn: Mental illness in the Islamic world pp.163–186. International Universities Press, Inc.

Bauman, Z (2000) Liquid Modernity. Polity Press, Cambridge.

BBC Radio 4 (2018) 'The Wrong Job: Square pegs in Round Holes' [online]. Available at https://www.bbc.co.uk/programmes/b0b88mgg (Accessed December 2020).

Beck, A (1967). Depression: Causes and treatment. Philadelphia: University of Pennsylvania Press.

Beck, A. T. (1976). Cognitive therapy and the emotional disorders. New York: International Universities Press.

Bergin, A, & Jensen, J (1990) Religiosity of psychotherapists: A national survey. Psychotherapy: Theory, Research, Practice, Training. 27(1), 3–7.

Bloom, W (2019) What is spiritual health? [online] At www.williambloom.com (Accessed December 2020).

Boadella, D (1987) Lifestreams: An introduction to biosynthesis. Routledge.

Boyton H (2014) The HEALTHY Group: A Mind–Body–Spirit Approach for Treating Anxiety and Depression in Youth. Journal of Religion & Spirituality in Social Work: Social Thought, 33:236–253.

Bradford Social Services/Bradford Community Health N.H.S. Trust/Bradford Interfaith Education Centre, (2001) Spiritual Well-being: Policy and Practice, Bradford.

Bragg, R, Wood, C and Barton, J (2013) Ecominds Effects on Mental Wellbeing; An Evaluation for MIND. [online]. London MIND. Available at: www.mind.org.uk/news-campaigns/campaigns/ecotherapy-works (Accessed December 2020).

Bronfenbrenner, U. (1979). The Ecology of Human Development: Experiments by Nature and Design. Cambridge, Massachusetts: Harvard University Press.

Burnham, J. (2012). Developments in Social GGRRAAACCEEESSS: visible-invisible, voiced-unvoiced. In I. Krause (Ed.), Cultural Reflexivity. London: Karnac.

Butler, Chapman, Forman, and Beck (2006). The empirical status of cognitive-behavioral therapy: A review of meta-analyses Clinical Psychology Review 26; 17 – 31.

Cain, S (2013) Quiet: The Power of Introverts in a World That Can't Stop Talking. Penguin.

Camden's black barbers - supermen in mental health battle (Feb 2016) [online]. London Camden CCG. Available at: www.camdenccg.nhs.uk/newsx (Accessed December 2020).

Campbell, J (2004) Pathways to Bliss: Mythology and Personal Transformation (Collected Works of Joseph). New World Library.

Christopherson, B (2020) [online]. The Increasing Population of the Spiritual but Not Religious — What Social Workers Need to Know. Available at: www.socialworktoday.com/news/pp_100517_2.shtml. (Accessed December 2020).

Clark, F (1973) Exploring intuition: Prospects and Possibilities Journal of Transpersonal Psychology, 5(2), 156-170.

Collins dictionary entry for spirit. Available at www.collinsdictionary.com/dictionary/english/spirit. (Accessed December 2020).

Collins, J (2001) Good To Great: Why Some Companies Make the Leap… and Others Don't. Random House Business.

Csikszentmihalyi M (2008). Flow: The Psychology of Optimal Experience. Harper Perennial modern classics.

Danylchuk (2015) What Do EMDR, Running, and Drumming Have in Common? [online]. Available at https://www.goodtherapy.org/blog/what-do-emdr-running-and-drumming-have-in-common-0901154. (Accessed December 2020).

Dein, S (2010) Religion, spirituality and mental health: theoretical and clinical perspectives Psychiatric Times 27(1) 28.

Dein, S, Cook, C, Powell, A, & Eagger, S. (2010) Religion, spirituality and mental health. The Psychiatrist, 34(2), 63-64.

De Mello, A (2011) Awareness: Conversations with the Masters. Crown Publishing Group.

Department of Health (2009) Religion or belief: A practical guide for the NHS. DH Publications.

D'Souza, R, Rich, D, Diamond, I, Godfery, K & Gleeson, D (2002) An open randomized control trial of a spiritually augmented cognitive behaviour therapy in patients with depression and hopelessness. Australian and New Zealand Journal of Psychiatry 36(6):A9.

Dummett, N (2006) Processes for Systemic Cognitive-Behavioural Therapy with Children, Young People and Families. Behavioural & Cognitive Psychotherapy 34(2); 179-189.

Ellis, A (1958) Rational psychotherapy. Journal of General Psychology, 59, 35–49.

Ellison, C (1983) Spiritual well-being: Conceptualization and measurement Journal of Theology and Psychology 11, 4.

Erikson, E (1959) Identity and the life cycle: Selected papers. Psychological Issues. 1: 1–171.

Erickson H (2007) Philosophy and theory of holism. Nursing Clinics of North America, 42, 139–163.

Fabry, J (1980) The Pursuit of Meaning. Harper & Row.

Fleury-Bahi, G, Pol, E & Navaro, O (2018) Handbook of Environmental Psychology and Quality of Life Research. Springer.

Frankl, V (1959) Man's Search for Meaning: The classic tribute to hope from the Holocaust. Rider (2004 edition).

Frazier, R, & Hansen, N (2009) Religious/spiritual psychotherapy behaviors: Do we do what we believe to be important? Professional Psychology: Research and Practice, 40(1), 81–87.

Garlick M, Wall K, Corwin D, Koopman C. (2011) Psycho-spiritual integrative therapy for women with primary breast cancer. Journal of Clinical Psychology in Medical Settings. 18(1):78-90.

Gendlin, E (1978) Focusing. New York, Everest House.

Gilbert, P (2009) Introducing compassion-focused therapy. Advances in Psychiatric Treatment, 15(3), 199-208.

Gilbert, P (2011) From the cradle – to beyond the grave? Quality in Ageing and Older Adults, 12 (3) 141-151.

Goddard, N.C. (1995) Spirituality as integrative energy: A philosophical analysis as requisite precursor to holistic nursing practice. Journal of Advanced Nursing. 22; 808-815.

Goldstein, W (2005) Defending the Human Spirit: Jewish Law's Vision for a Moral Society. Feldheim Pub.

Greenberger, D, & Padesky, C (1995). Mind over mood: A cognitive therapy treatment manual for clients. Guilford Press.

Hacker Hughes, J (2017). Towards a biopsychosociospiritual approach to psychological distress. Transpersonal Psychology Review 19(1), 13-15.

Hardy, A (1979) The spiritual nature of man: a study of contemporary religious experience. Oxford University Press.

Harris, R (2009) ACT Made Simple: An Easy-To-Read Primer on Acceptance and Commitment Therapy. Oakland, CA: New Harbinger.

Hayes S, Strosahl K, Wilson K (1999) Acceptance and Commitment Therapy: An Experiential Approach to Behavior Change. New York, NY: Guilford Press.

Heller, K (1989) The return to Community. American Journal of Community Psychology, 17, 1-16.

Hodge D (2006) Spiritually modified cognitive behavioural therapy: a review of the literature. Social Work 51, 157–166.

Hodge D (2008). Constructing spiritually modified interventions. International Social Work 51, 178–192.

James, W. (1890). The Principles of Psychology. New York, NY: H. Holt and Company.

James, A and Wells,A (2003) Religion and mental health: Towards a cognitive-behavioural framework British Journal of Health Psychology 8(3):359-76.

Jeffers, S (2007) Feel The Fear And Do It Anyway: How to Turn Your Fear and Indecision into Confidence and Action. Vermilion.

Johnson, R (1991) Inner Work: Using Dreams & Active Imagination for Personal Growth: Using Dreams and Active Imagination for Personal Growth. Harper San Francisco.

Jung, C (1933) Modern Man in Search of a Soul Translated by Dell, W & Baynes, C (2001) Routledge.

Jung, C (1966) Collected Works of C.G. Jung, Volume 7: Two Essays in Analytical Psychology. Princeton University Press.

Kellert, S (2018) Nature by Design: The Practice of Biophilic Design. Yale university press.

Kenny, A (1988) The Self. Marquette University Press.

Koenig, H, King, D, & Carson, V (2012) Handbook of religion and health (2nd ed.) Oxford University Press.

Laloux, F (2014) Reinventing Organizations: A Guide to Creating Organizations Inspired by the Next Stage in Human Consciousness. Nelson Parker.

Lazarus, A (1976) Multimodal behavior therapy: New York: Springer Pub. Co.

Levine, P (2010) In an Unspoken Voice: How the Body Releases Trauma and Restores Goodness. Berkeley, CA: North Atlantic Books.

Levoy, G (1997) Callings: Finding and Following an Authentic Life. Crown Publications.

Lewin, K (1951) Field Theory in Social Science. New York Harper.

Linehan M (1993) Cognitive-Behavioral Treatment of Borderline Personality Disorder. New York, NY: Guilford Press.

Lunden, O and Ulrich, R (1990) Effects of nature and abstract pictures on patients recovering from open heart surgery. Paper presented at the International Congress of Behavioural Medicine, 27-30 June Uppsala Sweden.

Martsolf, D., & Mickley, J. (1998). The concept of spirituality in nursing theories: Differing world-views and extent of focus. Journal of Advanced Nursing, 27, pp. 294–303.

Maslow, A (1954). Motivation and personality. Harpers.

Maslow, A (1971) The Farther Reaches of Human Nature. The Viking Press Inc., New York.

Masten, A, Cutuli, J, Herbers, J & Reed, M (2009). Resilience in development. In: Snyder, C & Lopez, S (Eds.) Oxford Handbook of Positive Psychology. 2nd ed. New York, NY: Oxford University Press.

McGeeney, A (2016) With Nature in Mind: The Ecotherapy manual for mental health professionals. Jessica Kingsley Publishers.

McGilchrist, I (2009) The Master and His Emissary: The Divided Brain and the Making of the Western World. Yale University Press.

McInnis E (2017) Black Psychology: A Paradigm for a Less Oppressive Clinical Psychology. Clinical Psychology Forum, 299, 3-8.

Mcleod, H and Ciarriochi, J (2012) The self in Cognitive Behavior therapy. In: McHugh, L and Stewart, I. (Eds.) The Self and Perspective-Taking: Theory and Research from Contextual Behavioral Science and Applied Approaches. pp.161-181. New Harbinger.

Merton, T (1962) New seeds of contemplation. New York New Directions.

Midlands Psychology Group (April 2014),Clinical Psychology Forum Special Issue; Draft Manifesto for a Social Materialist Psychology of Distress Clinical Psychology Forum. 256.

Mind over Mood - Aaron T. Beck Meets the Dalai Lama 2005 [online]. August 2012. Available at www.mindovermood.com/cbt-news/aaron-t-beck-meets-the-dalai-lama (Accessed December 2020).

Morrison, N (2001) Group cognitive therapy: Treatment of choice or sub-optimal option? Behavioural and Cognitive Psychotherapy, 29(3), 311–332.

Munroe, S and Steiner, S (1986) Social Support and psychopathology; interrelations with pre-existing disorder, stress and personality. Journal of Abnormal Psychology 95, 29-39.

Mulholland, H (2005) Counting on change Guardian 7th Dec.

Naeem, G, Ayub M, Kingdon D (2010) Psychologists experience of cognitive behaviour therapy in a developing country: a qualitative study from Pakistan. International Journal of Mental Health Systems. 28;4(1):2.

Ncube, N (2006) The Tree of Life Project: Using narrative ideas in work with vulnerable children in Southern Africa. The International Journal of Narrative Therapy and Community Work, 1, 3–16.

NHS England and NHS Improvement and the National Collaborating Central for Mental Health (2019) The Community Mental Health Framework for Adults and Older Adults. [online] Available at https://www.england.nhs.uk/publication/the-community-mental-health-framework-for-adults-and-older-adults/ (Accessed December 2020).

NHS England (2019). The NHS long term plan. [online] Available at https://www.longtermplan.nhs.uk/ (Accessed December 2020).

Norman, R (2018) Personal recording of National Spirituality and Mental Health Forum seminar on Atheism, spiritualty and mental health.

Ogden, P & Fisher, J (2014) Sensorimotor Psychotherapy: Interventions for Trauma and Attachment. W. W. Norton & Company.

Orford, J (1992) Community Psychology Theory and Practice. Wiley.

Otto, R (1923) The Idea of the Holy. Translated by Harvey, J. New York: Oxford University Press.

Padesky, C and Mooney, K (2012) Strengths-Based Cognitive–Behavioural Therapy: A Four-Step Model to Build Resilience. Clinical Psychology and Psychotherapy 19 (4) 283-290.

Paradis C, Friedman S, Lazar R, Grubea J (1996) Cognitive behavioral treatment of anxiety disorders in Orthodox Jews. Cognitive and Behavioral Practice 3, 271–288.

Pargament, K, Smith, B, Koenig, H, & Perez, L (1998). Patterns of positive and negative religious coping with major life stressors. Journal for the Scientific Study of Religion, 37, 71-725.

Pearce, W, (1976) The Co-ordinated Management of Meaning: A Rules-based Theory of Interpersonal Communication. In Miller, G.R. (Ed.), Explorations in Interpersonal Communication, pp. 17-36. Sage, Beverly Hills, CA.

Pennebaker, J & Smyth, J (2016) Opening Up by Writing It Down: How Expressive Writing Improves Health and Eases Emotional Pain. Guilford Press; 3rd edition.

Portnoy, G (1982). Where Everybody Knows Your Name Sung by Portnoy and Angelo.

Post B & Wade N (2009) Religion and spirituality in psychotherapy: a practice-friendly review of research. Journal of Clinical Psychology 65(2):131-46.

Propst L, Ostrom R, Watkins P, Dean T, Mashburn D (1992) Comparative efficacy of religious and nonreligious cognitive-behavior therapy for the treatment of clinical depression in religious individuals. Journal of Consulting and Clinical Psychology.;60:94–103.

Rath, T (2020) Life's Great Question: Discover How You Contribute To The World. Silicon Guild.

Rathod, S, Kingdon, D, Phiri, P & Gobbi, M (2010) Developing Culturally Sensitive Cognitive Behaviour Therapy for Psychosis for Ethnic Minority Patients by Exploration and Incorporation of Service Users' and Health Professionals' Views and Opinions. Behavioural and Cognitive Psychotherapy, 38 (5), 511–533.

Rogers, C (1951) Client Centred Therapy: Its Current Practice Constable & Co. Ltd.

Rohr, R (2011) Falling Upward: A Spirituality for the Two Halves of Life. Jossey-Bass.

Ross L (1997). Nurses' perceptions of spiritual care. Aldershot: Averbury.

Rotter, J (1966). Generalized expectancies for internal versus external control of reinforcement. Psychological Monographs, 80(1), 1–28.

Royal College of Psychiatrists (2006) Spirituality and mental health [online] Available at www.mentalhealth-media.org/uploads/3/0/1/9/30196951/rcp_spirituality_and_mh.pdf (Accessed December 2020).

Rowan, J (2005) The Transpersonal: Spirituality in Psychotherapy and Counselling. Routledge.

Sacks (2009) Succot is about the Resilience of the Human Spirit. [online] Available at https://rabbisacks.org/thought-for-the-day-2nd-october-2009-sukkot-is-about-the-resilience-of-the-human-spririt. (Accessed December 2020).

Sacks (2017) The Power of Ruach [online] Available at https://rabbisacks.org/power-ruach-beshalach-5777. (Accessed December 2020).

Segal Z, Williams J, & Teasdale J (2002). Mindfulness-based cognitive therapy for depression: A new approach to preventing relapse. New York, NY: Guilford Press

Seligman M (2002) Authentic Happiness: Using the New Positive Psychology to Realize Your Potential for Lasting Fulfillment. Random House Australia

Seligman M (2011) Flourish: A Visionary New Understanding of Happiness and Well-being. Simon & Schuster.

Siegel, D (2010) Mindsight: The New Science of Personal Transformation. Bantam Dell Pub Group.

Silf, M (1998) Landmarks: An Ignatian Journey: Exploration of Ignatian Spirituality. Darton, Longman & Todd Ltd.

Smuts J (1927) Holism and evolution. Macmillan and co. Ltd.

Spencer, S (2019) Think like a tree: The natural principles guide to life. Swarkestone Press.

Spitzer, R (1999) Patient Health Questionnaire : PHQ. New York State Psychiatric Institute.

Spitzer, R Kroenke, K Williams, J, Löwe, B (2006) A Brief Measure for Assessing Generalized Anxiety Disorder The GAD-7. Archives of Internal Medicine, 166(10):1092-1097.

Strawson, G (2017) The Subject of Experience. Oxford University Press.

Swinton, J (2001) Spirituality and mental health care. Jessica Kingsley Publishers.

Tajfel, H., Turner, J. C., Austin, W. G., & Worchel, S. (1979). An integrative theory of intergroup conflict. Organizational identity: A reader, 56-65.

Tedeschi, R & Calhoun, L (1995). Trauma & transformation: Growing in the aftermath of suffering. Sage Publications.

Tennant, R, Hiller, L, Fishwick, R, Platt, S, Joseph, S, Weich, S, Parkinson, J, Secker, J, & Stewart-Brown, S (2007) The Warwick-Edinburgh Mental Well-being Scale (WEMWBS): Development and UK validation. Health and Quality of Life Outcomes, 5, (63).

Thich Nhat Hanh (2015) Silence: The Power of Quiet in a World Full of Noise. Rider.

Tolle, E (1997) The Power of Now: A Guide to Spiritual Enlightenment. Namaste Press.

Tolle, E (2016) Stillness Speaks: Whispers of Now: A guide to spiritual enlightenment. Yellow Kite.

Tutu, D (2008) One Hour on CBC Interview. In Jolley, D (2011) [online] Available at www.suu.edu/hss/comm/masters/capstone/thesis/jolley-d.pdf. (Accessed December 2020).

Tutu, D [online] Available at www.goodreads.com/author/quotes/5943.Desmond_Tutu (Accessed December 2020).

Underhill, E (1937) The Spiritual Life. Four Broadcast Talks. London: Hodder & Stoughton.

Vaish, A, Grossmann, T & Woodward, A (2008) Not all emotions are created equal: The negativity bias in social-emotional development. Psychological Bulletin. 134(3): 383–403.

Vealey, R & Greenleaf, C (2006). Seeing is believing: Understanding and using imagery in sport. In: Williams, J.M. (Ed.), Applied Sport Psychology: Personal Growth to Peak Performance pp. 306-348. New York, NY: McGraw-Hill.

Waller, R, Trepka, C, Collerton, D, & Hawkins, J (2010) Addressing spirituality in CBT. The Cognitive Behaviour Therapist, 3(3), 95-106.

Walsh, R (2000) Essential Spirituality: The 7 Central Practices to Awaken Heart and Mind. John Wiley & Sons

Waterman (2014) Identity and Meaning: Contrasts of Existentialist and Essentialist Perspectives. International Journal of Existential Psychology and Psychotherapy Vol 5,1.

Weil, S (1949). The need for roots. Abingdon: Routledge Classics.

Wells, A & Matthews, G. (1994) Attention and emotion: A clinical perspective. Hove UK: Erlbaum (Psychology Press).

Wilber, K (2000) Integral Psychology: Consciousness, Spirit, Psychology, Therapy. Shambhala.

Wilber, K Patten, T Leonard, A & Morelli, M (2008) Integral Life Practice: A 21st Century Blueprint for Physical Health, Emotional Balance, Mental Clarity, and Spiritual Awakening. Integral Books.

Winnicott, D (1965) The Maturational Processes and the Facilitating Environment: Studies in the Theory of Emotional Development Karnac Books Ltd.

World Health Organization (2003) Investing in Mental Health. World Health Organization.

Yalom, I & Leszcz, M (1985). The Theory and Practice of Group Psychotherapy New York: Basic Books.

Yalom, I & Leszcz, M (2005). The Theory and Practice of Group Psychotherapy 5th edition. New York: Basic Books.

Young, J (1990). Practitioner's resource series. Cognitive therapy for personality disorders: A schema-focused approach. Professional Resource Exchange, Inc.

Zhang Y, Young D, Lee S, Li L, Zhang H, Xiao Z, Wei H, Feng Y, Zhou H, Chang D (2002) Chinese Taoist cognitive psychotherapy in the treatment of generalized anxiety disorder in contemporary China. Transcultural Psychiatry 39, 115–129.

Other titles from Pavilion Publishing

Free to be Me: A course manual to offer Holistic CBT as a group or individual therapy

Hilary Garraway (2021)

This course manual provides the guidance and resources needed to run a Holistic Cognitive Behaviour Therapy 'Free to be Me' course with individuals or groups, including clinical and non-clinical populations. It can be used therapeutically in any mental health and related setting, as well as in community and faith groups as a personal development course.

Therapy with a Map: A cognitive analytic approach to helping relationships

Steve Potter (2020)

The book gets to the heart of psychotherapy by exploring how core relational processes work regardless of model, and by presenting innovative techniques for using reflection, time and visual conversation maps to maximize effectiveness and improve client outcomes.

Working Effectively with Personality Disorder: Contemporary and critical approaches to clinical and organisational practice

Joanne Ramsden, Sharon Prince and Julia Blazdell (Eds) (2020)

The history of 'personality disorder' services is problematic to say the least. The very concept is under fire, services are often expensive and ineffective, and many service users report feeling that they have been deceived, stigmatised and excluded. Yet while there are, inevitably, serious (and often destructive) relational challenges involved in the work, creative networks of learning do exist – professionals who are striving to provide progressive, compassionate services for and with this client group.

Working Effectively with 'Personality Disorder' shares this knowledge, articulating an alternative way of working that acknowledges the contemporary debate around diagnosis, reveals flawed assumptions underlying current approaches, and argues for services that work more positively, more holistically and with a wider, more socially focused agenda.

The Acceptance and Commitment Therapy Diary: A guide and companion for moving toward the things that matter in your life

Dr Nic Hooper and Dr Freddy Jackson Brown (2021)

Life is often busy, demanding and full of challenges that can cause us to lose sight of what really matters. The Acceptance and Commitment Therapy (ACT) Journal is designed to help individuals to focus on the things that are most important to them by identifying personal values and putting them centre-stage where they can best guide actions and decisions.

Taking the form of a 12-week course of structured self-development, with ACT-informed guidance, reflection exercises, goal-setting tasks and inspirational quotations throughout, it is especially helpful for those currently engaged in ACT and other forms of brief therapy and/or coaching. However, the principles and lessons are relevant to anyone seeking to increase their personal well-being and build psychological flexibility – the ability to connect fully with experiences, including difficult thoughts and feelings, and pursue an authentic life.